DYSLEXIA

The Problem of Reading Retardation

DYSLEXIA

The Problem of Reading Retardation

T. S. HEPWORTH
B.A., Dip.Ed.(Q'ld.), Ed.D.(Harvard), M.A.C.E.
Lecturer in Education, Sydney Teachers' College

ST. MARTIN'S PRESS, NEW YORK

AFFILIATED PUBLISHERS: Macmillan & Company, Limited, London—
also at Bombay, Calcutta, Madras and Melbourne—The Macmillan
Company of Canada, Limited, Toronto

ACKNOWLEDGEMENTS

I wish to express my gratitude to my daughter, Mrs C. J. Sakidis, for the care and help she gave during the past decade to the many clients placed in her charge in the reading clinic which has been the basis for this book. Grateful parents will long remember her name.

Permission to include quotations and summaries from important books and learned articles is acknowledged in respect of *American Journal of Orthopsychiatry; Australian Journal of Psychology; British Medical Journal;* Cambridge University Press; The Johns Hopkins Press; *International Journal of Psychoanalysis* (Bailliere, Tindall & Cassell Ltd.); *Proceedings, Dyslexia Symposium,* Melbourne, 1968 (The Australian College of Speech Therapists); Munksgaard; *Journal of Genetic Psychology* (The Journal Press); William Heinemann Medical Books Ltd.; *The Slow Learning Child* (University of Queensland Press); *The Psychoanalytic Study of the Child.* The quoted sections are indicated where they occur in the text, by numbers referring to the bibliography where details are recorded in full.

Reference is also made to the Monograph, *Dyslexia,* by Dr A. Tomatis (translated by Dr A. Sidlauskas), University of Ottawa Press, 1969.

Mr John Hepworth took the photographs of Ingrid (Nos. 1 and 2), of Lisa (3 and 9) and of the clinic in operation (Mrs Sakidis and Mrs Ramsay; Nos. 5 and 8); No. 4 was made available by the United States Information Service; No. 6 by "Think Magazine"; No. 7 and the dust-jacket photograph by United Nations.

FOREWORD

Dr Hepworth has had a long practical experience in the diagnosis and treatment of reading disorders. In recent years he has been engaged with original research in dyslexia, which has elucidated some of the unsolved problems in reading retardation. These insights have thrown light on some of the difficult issues in dyslexia which have puzzled the most distinguished researchers for over a hundred years.

The present book is written in a style which is not overburdened with technical terms, and as such is a useful and much needed work which will be of assistance to speech therapists, reading therapists, educators, psychologists, and parents, and indeed anyone who has to deal with these kinds of problems.

Evan Davies, M.A. (Syd.), Ph.D. (N.S.W.)

CONTENTS

Photographs between pages 44 & 45.

PREFACE

On many occasions I have been called upon to lecture to various clubs and organisations on the subject of reading problems. Sometimes the request is to speak specifically on the topic of dyslexia, a term which is gaining currency and interest in the press, in professional circles—teachers, medical practitioners, psychologists —and amongst parents. Unfortunately, as will be demonstrated in the book, the term "dyslexia" is used either vaguely for reading difficulties generally, or by various writers in different ways, according to their professional background, or the school of thought to which they adhere.

For some time now I have been engaged in diagnostic and other remedial practice in this field, and at the same time have been carrying out research into dyslexia and other reading disabilities, my special interest being the effects of familial influence and emotional madadjustment on the problem. Additional to the analysis of hundreds of reading disability cases, this research has necessitated a close and extensive perusal of the professional literature concerning reading difficulties.

Obviously the detailed account of this research would have little practical value to any but advanced students working in a particular area of the field; but in view of the widespread interest I have indicated, it is timely that an outline, illustrating the various ways of looking at the matter, should be prepared. It would be useful to teachers, parents and students.

This, then, is the genesis of the present book; to outline the varying kinds of views as to the causes of reading disabilities, to ask whether there is a specific kind of reading disability, severer than the other kinds, perhaps, that might be labelled "dyslexia" (a term which in essence implies simply "difficulty with words"), and to indicate some ways that have been suggested for diagnosing and dealing with such difficulties.

To do this I have indicated some of the representative thinking about the problem by psychologists and educationalists, psycho-

analysts and neurologists; and to illustrate better the stand they
have adopted, I have included case material showing ways in
which some of the workers in this field have applied their theories
to diagnosis and treatment of particular cases.

Parents and teachers, when confronted with reading disability
in a child, are naturally concerned to ask the question:
"Can this child be helped to read with less difficulty?"

I believe the answer to this question in almost every case is
"yes", and some space has been set aside for discussion of it—
apart from the reference to treatments that have come up in relation to outlines of theories, in various chapters.

Nevertheless, the book does not set itself up as a manual or
"do-it-yourself" kit for remedial reading. Its main purpose is the
discussion and illustration of *viewpoints,* with the hope that some
readers will be impelled to further thinking about this problem;
and to assist them in doing this, a comprehensive bibliography is
included at the end. It must not be assumed that, because a particular point of view is outlined in the book, this necessarily represents
my support for it, or my belief in its validity. The fact that the
problem of dyslexia is seen so differently by well-known writers
and researchers in this field should strike a note of caution against
the temptation to oversimplify the problem and to see it only in
one particular way.

It is for this reason that my own support would be mainly for
the sentiments expressed in Chapter 5, where it is suggested that
severe reading disability may arise from many different causes, so
that we may have, for example, social, cultural or educational
dyslexia, depending on the circumstances and origin of any particular case. No doubt the use of these adjectives (and others) applied
to dyslexia will be disputed by some who prefer a one-cause
approach and a specific (but, I believe, hard to substantiate)
meaning for the term. However, I consider that these are useful,
descriptive concepts that will be readily understood.

The inclusion of these schools of thought has, of course, a value
additional to the illustration of varied ways of thinking about
dyslexia. One does not have to be an outright adherent to the
psychoanalytic school, for example, to see validity in the claim
that the formative early years are (or, as I see it, *may* be) important in shaping the kind of reader, or person, that a child will
become. Similarly, we may be very concerned about the part
environmental factors play in the area of reading difficulties, while

at the same time prepared to concede the possibility, or probability, of hereditary influence in some cases. So each school of thought, if not interpreted too rigidly, may shed some light on the problem, differing, perhaps, in emphasis from case to case.

Finally, a word about terminology. All disciplines have their jargon, and psychology is no exception to this. I have endeavoured to avoid over-use of technical terms, but at the same time a serious reader deserves to be treated seriously—certainly not to be spoken down to. Psychological terms have therefore been used where it was felt that clarity would suffer by substitution.

A year appearing in brackets after an author's work refers to an entry in the bibliography. For example, Vernon (1967) refers to Vernon's publication listed with that date. Thus footnotes have been kept to a minimum.

T. S. HEPWORTH
Sydney, 1971

1

THE HISTORY AND NATURE OF THE PROBLEM

Tucked away inconspicuously in *The British Medical Journal* of November 7, 1896, between an article on "Dermatitis Caused by Roentgen X-Rays" and another on "Filiaris in Samoa" is a report by a medical practitioner in Seaford, Sussex, England, W. Pringle Morgan, which was destined to stand as a landmark in our attempt to understand and deal with the strange phenomenon of a supposedly literate society—the fact that scattered here and there, in city and country, in well-to-do suburbs and in those not so well-to-do, among people of average and above average (even high) intelligence, there are those who, though exposed to the written word at school, on hoardings and on railway stations, cannot read, or if they are able to read a little, do so only with the greatest of difficulty.

This is what Dr Morgan had to say:

A CASE OF CONGENITAL WORD BLINDNESS

Percy F.—a well-grown lad, aged 14—is the eldest son of intelligent parents, the second child of a family of seven. He has always been a bright intelligent boy, quick at games, and in no way inferior to others of his age.

His greatest difficulty has been—and is now—his inability to learn to read. This inability is so remarkable, and so pronounced, that I have no doubt it is due to some congenital defect.

He has been at school or under tutors since he was 7 years old, and the greatest efforts have been made to teach him to read, but in spite of this laborious and persistent training, he can only wtih difficulty spell out words of one syllable.

The following is the result of an examination I made a short time since. He knows all his letters, and can write them and read them. In writing from dictation he comes to grief over any but the simplest words. For instance, I dictated the following sentence: "Now, you watch me while I spin it". He wrote: "Now you word me wale I spin it"; and again: "Carefully winding the string round the peg", was written: "Calfuly winder the sturng rond the Pag".

In writing his own name he made a mistake, putting "Precy" for "Percy", and he did not notice the mistake until his attention was called to it more than once. I asked him to write the following words:

Song	..	..	..	..	..	.. he wrote	.. ..	scone
Subject	..	..	..	..	..	„	.. ..	scojock
Without	.	..	..	..	..	„	.. ..	wichout
English	.	..	..	..	..	„	.. ..	Englis
Shilling	.	..	..	..	..	„	.. ..	sening
Seashore		..	..	..	..	„	.. ..	seasow

He was quite unable to spell the name of his father's house, though he must have seen it and spelt it scores of times. On asking him to read the sentences he had just written a short time previously he could not do so, but made mistakes over every word except the simplest. Words such as "and" and "the" he always recognises.

I then asked him to read me a sentence of an easy child's book without spelling the words. The result was curious. He did not read a single word correctly, with the exception of "and", "the", "of", "that", etc.; the other words seemed to be quite unknown to him, and he could not even make an attempt to pronounce them.

I next tried his ability to read figures, and found he could do so easily. He read off quickly the following: 785,852,017; 20,969; and worked out correctly: $(a + x) (a - x) = a^2 - x^2$. He could not do the simple calculation $4 \times \frac{1}{2}$, but he multiplied 749 by 867 quickly and correctly. He says he is fond of arithmetic, and finds no difficulty with it, but that printed or written words "have no meaning to him", and my examination of him quite convinces me that he is correct in that opinion. Words written or printed seem to convey no impression to his mind, and it is only after laboriously spelling them that he is able, by the sounds of the letters, to discover their import. His memory for written or printed words is so defective that he can only recognise such simple ones as "and", "the", "of", etc. Other words he never seems to remember, no matter how frequently he may have met them.

He seems to have no power of preserving and storing up the visual impression produced by words—hence the words, though seen, have no significance for him. His visual memory for words is defective or absent; which is equivalent to saying that he is what Kussmaul has termed "word blind"[1] (*caecitas syllabaris et verbalis*).

Cases of word blindness are always interesting, and this case is, I think, particularly so. It is unique, so far as I know, in that it follows upon no injury or illness, but is evidently congenital, and due most

---

[1] See footnote 2 page 6.

probably to defective development of that region of the brain, disease of which in adults produces practically the same symptoms—that is, the left angular gyrus.

I may add that the boy is bright and of average intelligence in conversation. His eyes are normal, there is no hemianopsia, and his eyesight is good. The schoolmaster who has taught him for some years says that he would be the smartest lad in the school if the instruction were entirely oral. It will be interesting to see what effect further training will have on his condition.

His father informs me that the greatest difficulty was found in teaching the boy his letters, and they thought he would never learn them. No doubt he was originally letter blind (*caecitas litteralis*), but by dint of constant application this defect has been overcome.

The Incidence of Reading Retardation

Before going on to discuss the nature of "word-blindness", or "dyslexia", or "reading disability", and whether or not these terms refer to one problem, or to several different problems, or sometimes to one problem and sometimes to another, we may note estimates given by experts as to the widespread incidence of reading difficulties. The most extensive surveys have been carried out in the United States, but some estimates have been made also in Australia and the United Kingdom and elsewhere; the estimates vary quite a deal, but they all leave us with the uncomfortable feeling that there are more reading casualties in the community than most people would imagine. Here are two statements from America that the author believes from experience might very well apply to Australia:

1. According to figures quoted (1960) by the *Dyslexia Memorial Institute,* associated with the Wesley Hospital, Chicago, about 30 per cent of the pupils in grades four, five and six show that they do not have sufficient reading proficiency to handle the programme of the typical American Elementary School.

2. *Dr James Bryant Conant,* formerly President of Harvard University, states that, after carrying out a survey of American Secondary Education under the auspices of the Carnegie Foundation, he has come to the conclusion that 40 per cent of pupils in the first, second and third years of American High Schools are reading at the Sixth Grade level, or less.

Surveys that I have carried out with large numbers of pupils in Australian schools would tend to support these views, providing a reasonably wide definition of reading disability is allowed.

Definition

It is appropriate at this point to look at some of the definitions of dyslexia and reading disability used by various writers, and some of the yardsticks employed to carry out diagnoses in various instances.

In the School Surveys, for instance, carried out by the author and referred to above, a pupil was regarded as manifesting reading disability in *some* measure, however slight, if he failed to score at least a "C" score (eighth centile rank) on a scaling from "A+" down to "E—" for the month and the year of his school grade. For example, if all 5th class children in a school were being tested, in March, the pupil would be expected to score at least at the eighth centile rank for March of 5th class in the State concerned (New South Wales in this case) in all three reading level tests employed (A.C.E.R. Form "C" Parts 1, 2 and 3, namely Word Recognition, Speed and Reading for Meaning), or be noted as below the expected level. Obviously this covered a fair range of "retardation" as some pupils so labelled may have failed to score the expected minimum in one area or test only, while others may have failed to reach the minimum level in two or three parts of the tests; again, some may have failed to reach the minimum level by a narrow margin only, others by a wide margin, and so on.

Obviously, while this was a useful criterion and sorted the pupils quickly into two groups—those who reached the expected minimum level in all areas, and those who did not in at least one area, other criteria now had to be used pupil by pupil; thus a pupil below the arbitrary cut-off point for the grade and month, even perhaps by a wide margin and maybe in all three tests, might nevertheless be working up to his personal ceiling, while another who *did* score *at or even above* the minimum required level, might not be measuring up to his own level. In other words, the presence or absence of a "gap" between ability and performance is the crucial factor in deciding whether or not a pupil is in need of remedial assistance; it is not, however, the crucial factor in deciding whether or not a particular pupil has (to use the expression in the Dyslexia Institute statement referred to earlier) "sufficient reading proficiency to handle the programme of the typical elementary school (or grade)".

In point of fact, however, most of the low scorers in the reading tests do show a gap between ability and performance—the number of low scorers not manifesting such a gap—that is, those whose

low scores are solely attributable to low ability—are relatively few
in number.

A count of failure to reach the pre-determined cut-off point
(the "C" level) in at least one test, normally gives a number of
about 25 in 110 pupils—something of the order mentioned in the
Institute Survey.

DYSLEXIA

This is not to say that the 20 to 25 per cent of children in the
5th classes tested by the author can be diagnosed as "suffering
from" or "having" dyslexia, for two reasons: firstly, because many
of the 20 to 25 per cent are cases of relatively mild reading retardation, while the term "dyslexia" is normally reserved for quite
severe cases; secondly, even with the severe cases, there is, as noted
in the preface, disagreemnt amongst the "experts" as to the exact
meaning of the term "dyslexia", some insisting that it is best used
to describe, by differential diagnosis, a specific syndrome, others
that it covers a variety of severe reading problems, which I suppose
might be referred to as dyslexia $(_1)$, dyslexia $(_2)$, dyslexia $(_3)$, and
so on, depending on special symptoms, varying causal factors, and
other distinguishing characteristics in each case.

Most of the proponents of these varying viewpoints have specific
theories, psychological, physiological, neurological, educational,
etc., on which their definitions of dyslexia or reading disability
rest; one gets the feeling, at least with some of the theorists, that
they are carrying particular chips on their shoulders, are irritated
by other suggested aetiological or causative factors and are bent
on defending the particular theories they support.

One way of illustrating this situation is to instance some of the
major theories and/or definitions put forward by prominent
researchers with some of their case material quoted by way of
elaboration. But it has already been made clear that I have not
found it necessary to ally myself dogmatically with any one theory
to the exclusion of all others, in conducting satisfactorily a Reading
Disability and Dyslexia Clinic, but incline more to a broader point
of view, finding worthwhile contributions in a number of theories,
some of which fit certain clients more readily than others, and
certainly accept the (to me) proven fact of multiple causation in
some cases and more specific causation in others. I doubt that a
really strong case has been made out by the proponents of specific
or developmental dyslexia in the sense in which certain neurologists (especially Critchley, 1964, as we shall see) use these terms.

One is left with the feeling at times that, as a final resort, the neurologists, when faced with a decision as to whether a patient exhibiting a severe reading disability, and known to be neither a brain-damaged victim, nor a mental defective, nor a person having a history of severe illness or accident, will say, "I *know* that this is a case of developmental dyslexia, congenitally determined and not a case of reading disability, no matter how severe, of some other kind", but somehow not support the unequivocal diagnosis with evidence, at least to the satisfaction of the present author.

All researchers and theorists who use the term dyslexia, or perhaps congenital word blindness,[2] are talking of a syndrome or syndromes—that is, a group or groups of symptoms—characterized by an apparent inability to learn to read, at least by normal methods, even though the individual may possess intelligence of normal or superior level; indeed non-reading by mental defectives or severely brain-damaged victims, where a very low ceiling of possible attainment (almost nil perhaps) may operate, is a special problem very different from those we are considering. They are talking of non-readers of average or even high intelligence who yet cannot read—as in the case quoted earlier by Dr Pringle Morgan—and surprise people by the fact that they cannot do so. Those of us closely connected with this field are indeed impressed with the number of cases who come to a Dyslexia or Reading Disability Clinic who not only appear bright, and often achieve satisfactorily or highly in certain other school subjects—say arithmetic—or even in some instances manage firms and businesses quite well—but also score satisfactorily or at a high level on tests of intelligence. Such tests would, of course, be non-verbal intelligence tests (puzzle-solving tests) or individually administered tests where reading questions do not form an important part of the test.

Schools of Thought

The following are some of the major and more interesting theories that have been put forward to explain the strange pheno-

---

[2] The expression "word blindness", once popular and still found in some clinic names, such as the Word Blind Centres in London and Copenhagen and elsewhere, is falling into disuse. The dyslexic child *can* see words, but for him some words and letter shapes do not have perceptual constancy—that is, they are perceived differently in different phrases or sentences and in differing positions.

menon of severe reading retardation. They can be grouped as follows:

> Neurological-congenital theories.
> Other theories emphasising the hereditary concept.
> Psychoanalytically-based theories.
> Theories emphasising emotional factors derived from environmental experience.
> Theories that suggest multiple causation and the possibility of various "kinds" of dyslexia.

This has been well put, in another way, by Dr Abraham Fabian, Director of the Brooklyn Juvenile Center, New York. In a paper published in the *American Journal of Orthopsychiatry*, 1955, he writes:

Reading disability, so ubiquitous a symptom of childhood, has attracted specialists from many fields of investigation, including several branches of medicine, psychology and pedagogy. Out of the multidisciplinary approaches have arisen divergent opinions on several aspects of the problem. The many theories on aetiology that have been proposed in the past 75 years of research on reading retardation can be grouped under the following three headings: organ-centred, school-centred and child-centred, the last category referring particularly to emotional problems underlying learning difficulties. [Fabian adds that to these must be added a fourth category—family-centred.] Massive chronic familial psychopathology, aside from its influence aetiologically, has significant prognostic and therapeutic implications in reading disability.

In other words, not only are there numerous "reading casualties" in the one family, or related families, in many cases, thus pointing to heredity as the "cause" in such cases, but the prospect of helping individuals from those families would, he feels, be influenced by this heredity factor.

Fabian goes on to elaborate his summary. By *organ-centred* theories, he means those theories which take into account problems of vision and hearing and touch and neurological factors which are part of our physical make-up.

School-centred

Some reading problems, severe and mild, seem to stem from experiences in the early school life of the child; poor teaching; over-crowded classes, to mention two possibilities. Some see emotional problems developing along with the reading problems at school, others feel that unless the emotional problems were already there, the reading difficulties would mostly not arise despite unfortunate school experiences. We must allow, too, for the frequent *build-up* of emotional problems as a result of reading difficulties, whether or not we agree that the emotional problems commenced as a result of the reading difficulties. The educators, says Fabian, not unnaturally welcomed the physical (organ-centred) theories, but in the long run found such theories unsupported by surveys and by the teacher's day-to-day experience of reading problems. But they have been "reluctant to attribute reading retardation solely to inadequate teaching programmes".

Child-centred

Here, Fabian has in mind the psychoanalysts or psychoanalytically trained observers. They put forward dynamic considerations "ranging from diffuse blocks in children with pleasure-ridden personalities who cannot tolerate the frustration that attends learning, to specific inhibitions stemming from particular phantasies".

There is no doubt that if you want quotations that will make you "sit up" and take notice, the psychoanalysts—or those who write about them—have some that must surely be unbeatable. Thus Fabian—still on reading problems and their causes: "When phallic stirrings arouse excessive castration fears there may be interference with competitive efforts and mastery. Defensive struggles against scotophilia may discourage curiosity and compromise epistemophilic drives." (If you do not fully understand this suggestion or its implication to reading, do not be unduly concerned—there are many people, including several who are dealing successfully with reading problems, who are in much the same boat as you are.)

Family-centred

There is quite a deal of evidence that reading problem *families*— perhaps stretching back several generations—exist. Later we shall discuss this in more detail, especially as it relates to an important Scandinavian study carried out twenty years ago (Hallgren, 1950). But while it is true that the pupil "brings his family to school", and all his family background, some at least of this "familial influence" on his reading success or failure must be attributable to the environment of the family as well as to the familial genes.

What Fabian has sought to demonstrate is his hypothesis that *reading disability is an index to pathology*—in short, by the form taken by a reading disability in an individual, a group or a family, we have clues, or an index, to the pathology (emotional and perhaps physical) that has shaped the disability and caused it to come into being.

Another summary that again highlights various types of theories and alleged causative factors that have been put forward to explain the incidence of dyslexia, is one by Arthur Gates, 29 years ago, in the *Journal of Genetic Psychology,* who writes:

In their attitude toward the role of personality maladjustment in reading disability, specialists in remedial reading could be found at all steps between two extremes. At the one extreme are specialists who think that personality factors and adjustments are so rarely the causes of reading difficulty (although they may often be the result) as to make extensive investigation of personality factors futile. At the other extreme are persons who consider that most, if not all, reading disabilities are merely one symptom of a deep-seated general maladjustment. According to the former, emotional distress is cured by teaching the child to read; according to the latter, the child's reading defect is cured by removing the emotional distress. Between these two extremes are many other views. Some hold that emotional maladjustment and reading defects are concomitant, neither causing the other. Some hold that the one is sometimes cause, sometimes effect, sometimes concomitant.

In other words, given the existence of a reading problem in an individual, and given also perhaps (very likely, in my view) the existence in the same individual, *at the same time,* of an emotional, tension-like, personality-type problem, is one the cause of the other —and if so, which of the two is the cause and which the effect? Or are both the outcome of some third, earlier causal factor, such as a congenital problem transmitted through the genes or, as the psychoanalytical school would hold, a probable interference in the first months of life, with the normal course of psycho-sexual development? And so on.

It is obvious from all this that there is a considerable, perhaps bewildering, range of possible ætiology or causative factors to choose from; but the bewilderment lessens if we bear in mind the view held by many sound researchers in this field—the "many-causes" view, each cause leading perhaps to a more or less specific syndrome or group of symptoms or type of dyslexia or reading difficulty.

It is important to stress again that adherence to a particular line of thinking or school of thought is not an essential prerequisite to the successful treatment of reading problems.

VARYING RESPONSES TO THE SAME STIMULI

As a point of interest, Gates reminds us of the difficulty we may have in either searching *back* to a specific cause or *looking forward* to probable outcomes of an existing present set of circumstances in the life of a child, if we note the very different reactions to the "same" stimulus by two individuals. This can be noted readily when a child puts his philosophy into words. For example:

Child A: "I won't do anything that that girl likes to do".

Child B: "I'll do better than Bill if it kills me".

John Money, in *The Disabled Reader* (Ed.), 1967, in discussing the topic, "On Learning and Not Learning to Read", summarizes what he calls "the impediments to learning". He agrees that they arise from many sources and says that this applies to the "learning of school subjects in general or of reading in particular". As specific impediments he instances deficient vision or hearing; or as examples of more general factors, chronic debility or mental deficiency. The wide divergencies range from "localised malfunction of, or injury to, the brain" to "learning blocks arising out of the life history of the individual". He includes genetic factors, as well as physical injury to the developing embryo, or traumatic injury at birth. Infections or traumatic experiences after birth may occur and have an adverse effect, and so may lack of exposure at the critical time "to the proper experiential stimulation" necessary for the development of adequate language skills.[3] At a later stage the factor of inadequate teaching may interfere with this development. Important, too, are the standards of the family and community of which the child forms part, and which, in some areas, may be tolerant towards incomplete schooling. Then again, the attitudes of other boys and girls of the same age are important. "The ideals and traditions of the peer group may . . . put no premium on academic survival, so that to be a 'big shot' means to have achieved status as a non-learner and perhaps to be a graduate in delinquency, as well."

---

[3] He refers to this as "behavioural and linguistic growth and differentiation".

2

DYSLEXIA AND THE FAMILY TREE

It has been interesting to note in dealing with the cases of reading disability that have passed through my own clinic, how often one encounters "familial instances"—that is, individuals from the one family seeking assistance for a reading problem. Sometimes (in fact in perhaps almost 40 per cent of the cases) two or more siblings are receiving help at the same time or at different times. Cousins, too, are seen, though less frequently. Sometimes when questioning a parent during the interview as to number, ages and school progress (or lack of it) of the children in the family, the parent will say about an older brother or sister of the child brought for testing: "He was just the same. I wish I had known of how to get help for him at the time". Or about a younger child: "She's starting off just like her brother [the present client] did".

At other times, although our interview questionnaire has not included detailed questions about generations prior to the child being tested, apart from a simple question as to whether the mother and father like reading, information is often forthcoming to the effect that "I had the same difficulty myself; still do in fact"; or "her father has never been a 'good' reader; says he always had trouble with it". One mother stated recently about a daughter: "Her father says it is history repeating itself. He was a very poor reader at school—is still hesitant—and his father, before him, was just as bad."

Perhaps the gem of all such quotations was a statement made to me recently in an interview by a medical practitioner who had brought her son along for diagnostic appraisal: "You know this dyslexia thing—he had it a bit, so did I, and other members of the family".

It must be admitted at once that this is not statistical evidence—

but it leaves a very definite impression on the mind of the clinician. But, as already mentioned, the possible influence of environment on the behaviour of a child cannot be set dogmatically aside, even when heredity seems to be the most logical explanation, for environment includes family environment.

On the other hand, in at least some studies, reference is made to the appearance of what seems to be the same syndrome in sets of twins. This, again, is a line of investigation that can be misleading, for twins will share the "same" environment more "exactly" than ordinary siblings. To my mind, however, it is a line of thinking which is, to say the least, highly suggestive.

Before passing on to further discussion of familial instances, it might be mentioned that in our clinic we have had a family group of three sons of the one father—two to a first wife, now divorced, one to a second wife. In both cases the mothers concerned came along for interview and were quite different personalities in the interviewing situation.

Here again we have nothing of absolute proof, but a definitely interesting situation which one is tempted to take at its face value. Certainly the chance of environmental influence is lower than in the case of brothers or sisters born of the same father and mother and reared by them, and much lower than in the case of twins— whether "identical" or "fraternal".

Bertil Hallgren

Not a great deal of research has been reported in connection with heredity and dyslexia, although reference to it (for and against) has appeared in many works. One study, however, that is well-known in this connection was carried out by a physician, Bertil Hallgren, at the Psychiatric Clinic at Karolinska Institutet during the years 1947-50.

Hallgren's method of investigation was to carry out a detailed case-study procedure with extensive diagnostic testing sessions and interviewing of subjects.

He studied cases both of whose parents were dyslexic; dyslexics with one dyslexic parent only; cases where neither of the parents was dyslexic, but where the syndrome had appeared in uncles, aunts, great-uncles or great-aunts.

Hallgren makes it quite clear that he regards "Specific Dyslexia" or "Congenital Word Blindness" as a particular kind of disability, differentiated from other varieties of reading disabilities (such as the reading disability that may follow a brain injury) and occurring in subjects predisposed by heredity to fall a victim to it.

PRIMARY AND SECONDARY DISABILITIES

He tries to make a clear distinction between *primary* reading disabilities (that is, the type passed on through the genes) and *secondary* (that is, the type or types that arise as a result of physical, mental or environmental factors after birth—e.g., illness, cerebral disorders, visual and auditory defects, speech defects, disturbances in hand or eye dominance, mental subnormality, mental illness or emotional disorders, adverse school or home conditions, and so on).

On the face of it, the distinction he is drawing between the two kinds of reading disabilities is pretty clear cut, but he is far less convincing as to the possibility, let alone probability, of determining, for a particular patient, the category to which he belongs.

In selecting his cases for study, Hallgren laid down for himself the following diagnostic criteria:

1. Difficulties in learning to read and write;
2. Proficiency in reading and writing during the first years at school definitely below the average of the class the child attended;
3. A definite discrepancy between proficiency in reading and writing and in other school subjects;
4. A definite discrepancy between proficiency in reading and writing and the child's general intelligence.

The neurologists, who would be unlikely to argue with the above criteria, would press also for a long and *detailed* physical examination, with a neurologist present.

Many children in our clinic would fit some of the above symptomatology, while some would fit all of it, but I would by no means regard them all (or even many of them) as dyslexic in the specific sense indicated by Hallgren.

In carrying out his diagnosis, Hallgren used case histories, school reports, statements by the subject and others, and tests made up by himself, which were not standardized.

At any rate, whether Hallgren or anyone else has succeeded in making out a case for specific dyslexia of congenital origin, or not, is not very important. He has drawn our attention to the manifestation or occurrence of severe reading disability in members of family groups. This has added support to the belief that others have held, that familial instances are of at least fairly frequent occurrence.

For those with an interest in genetics, Hallgren's summary of his findings is quoted:

"The genetic-statistical analysis shows that specific dyslexia, with a high degree of probability, follows a monohybrid autosomal mode of inheritance." This means, among other things, that it is carried on *autosomes* (that is, chromosomes other than sex chromosomes). He was not sure, however, whether heredity played a part in certain of his cases, and if it did play a part, to what extent.

In other words, while Hallgren was firmly convinced that dyslexia was a quite specific problem which would be discovered by careful diagnosis, in practice he found this difficult to do. So he agrees that it would seem that in the cases he finally did select for his study, "there is no sharp borderline between the group of cases of specific dyslexia and the group of other cases".

It seems to the author that Hallgren fell back on this admission as a convenient (but sincere) explanation of apparent anomalies in those instances where individuals did not seem to fall readily into the hereditary pattern—they *must* have been undetected cases of "secondary" reading disability, because if they had been "primary cases" they *would* have fitted into the pattern. In short, if a case is made out for something and some instances turn up that seem to be contrary to it, they are set aside as probably "different", and so the case remains undisturbed.

I have mentioned that many authors have referred to the possibility or probability of the operation of heredity in reading problems. Their writings go back at least to the first years of the present century and earlier. There was fairly wide acceptance of the belief that direct inheritance could be shown to operate in two generations, while some researchers (e.g., Marshall and Ferguson, 1939) found evidence (to their satisfaction) of congenital influence in three generations and a few (e.g., Skydsgaard, 1942 and Hallgren himself) in four generations or more.

The Study of Twins

There is no question in my mind, after years of experience with cases of reading disability, that such problems do *tend* to run in families (with twin cases, among others, in our files) and I am highly suspicious that this family influence is at least partially of an hereditary nature.

The study of twins, especially monozygotic, identical twins, is always interesting. The Mendelian laws of inheritance would lead us to expect that if dyslexia is genetically determined, and one twin in a pair of identical twins is found to be affected by it, the other twin will also be found to be so affected, and that this will hold true for 100 per cent of cases. If, on the other hand, the twins are dizygotic, or fraternal, the chance that the second twin will be so affected is similar to the position with two siblings in general, namely the probability is 50 per cent, if the mode of inheritance is monohybrid autosomal dominant, and one parent only carries an infected inheritance.

The literature on dyslexia carries relatively few reports of studies on twins, but there are some and where the twins concerned were monozygotic, Hallgren claims that the expectancies as to inheritance seem to be fulfilled.

But there still remains the serious trap we have mentioned in twin studies—that twins (and especially identical twins) share a very close environmental relationship which might very well increase the possibility of environmental influence, giving the appearance of heredity. And, again, where this principle does not seem to be operating it could again be assumed that we have in fact a case of "secondary" reading disability, mistakenly diagnosed as specific dyslexia.

In Hallgren's study there were four pairs of twins and he included two other pairs in his report on twins. He notes also that one of the "affected" parents (mother) of one of his subjects was a twin. The history of her twin brother suggested that a diagnosis of specific dyslexia could be made, but as it was not possible to examine the brother personally, this pair of twins was omitted from the report.

There were therefore six pairs of twins—twelve subjects—in the first analysis, not a large number or even a sufficient number to pronounce upon with any degree of statistical certainty, but again interesting and suggestive.

The first task was to determine whether or not the twins in each pair were monozygotic or dizygotic. If they fulfilled the following criteria they were classified as monozygotic:

1. They were of the same sex.
2. They looked so alike that they were hard to tell from one another.
3. The colour and structure of their irises were essentially similar.
4. The colour and texture of the hair were essentially similar.

5. Skin colour in each twin of a pair was the same, and where freckles were present, there was the same number of them and they were distributed in the same way.

6. The shape of the ears (in detail) was the same.

7. Size and shape of lips and shape of nose were essentially the same.

8. Very importantly—the blood group combination was the same.

Applying this criteria, Hallgren classified three of his six pairs of twins as monozygotic; the other three pairs were dizygotic—no special criteria had to be applied with these—they were opposite sex twins.

THE DIZYGOTIC TWINS

Pair 1: Nine years old at the time of examination. Parents were both affected and one brother also. The mother was diagnosed "borderline case"—that is, *possibly* suffering from secondary reading disability.

One twin (girl) in this pair was diagnosed as a moderately severe case of specific dyslexia; I.Q. 100, nail-biter; right-handed.

The other twin (boy) showed no signs of specific dyslexia; I.Q. 109; nail-biter; right-handed.

Pair 2: Nine years old. The mother and one brother were "affected", the father was not. That is, the parent mating was "affected" X "unaffected".

Both twins in this pair showed signs of slight specific dyslexia. The boy obtained an I.Q. rating of 113, was a nail-biter and regarded as a "problem child" with a regressive personality. The girl obtained an I.Q. rating of 128.

Pair 3: Nine years old. Parent mating was "affected" (mother) X "unaffected" (father). One sister was also affected.

The boy was diagnosed as a case of moderately severe specific dyslexia. His I.Q. rating was 129. Enuretic. Classified as a "regressive-type problem child". Left-handed.

The girl showed no signs of specific dyslexia and although an intelligence test was not administered to her, her papers were noted "intelligence apparently good". Right-handed.

THE MONOZYGOTIC TWINS

Pair 4: (Boys) eleven years old. Both were colour-blind. Parent mating was "affected" X "unaffected". The mother (diagnosed "borderline case") was the affected parent; one brother of the twins was also diagnosed as a case of specific dyslexia.

Both twins were classified "moderately severe" dyslexics; one obtained an I.Q. rating of 113, the other of 106 (in this latter case the I.Q. test was not continued to the "higher level".

Forceps birth for both twins. One only was left-handed.

Pair 5: (Girls) twelve years old. Same blood group. Parent mating was "affected" (father) X "unaffected". Father was denoted "borderline case" because he had learned to compensate for his problem to the point where diagnosis was rendered more difficult; one of the father's sister's daughters was regarded as suffering probably from specific dyslexia.

One of the twins obtained an I.Q. rating of 104, the other of 114. Instrumental (forceps) delivery in the one case (I.Q. 104) and normal birth in the other. Both were diagnosed as "slight" specific dyslexics. Development after birth was normal, but both were nail-biters and both suffered from eczema at the fold of the elbows and palms of the hands. Both were right-handed. One twin (I.Q. 114) showed transient stuttering at age 3-4; the other exhibited no speech defect.

Pair 6: (Girls) ten years old. Parent mating "affected" (father) X "unaffected" (mother). One of the father's brothers was left-handed, stuttered as a child and was reported to have had difficulty with arithmetic. Another of the father's brothers also stuttered as a child.

The twins were both diagnosed as cases of "moderately severe specific dyslexia". I.Q. ratings were 114 and 116. Normal births. Normal development. Both were right-handed, but in one (I.Q. 116) there was a tendency to left-handedness earlier.

Hallgren summarizes his study of these six pairs of twins as follows:

The analysis thus shows that, of the three dizygotic pairs of twins, one was concordant and two were discordant with respect to specific dyslexia. All three monozygotic pairs of twins were concordant in this respect. The results are in agreement with the hypothesis that specific dyslexia is genetically conditioned.

He agrees however that the number of pairs of twins studied is small and warns against drawing absolute conclusions from this.

concordant→constant.

3

DELVING INTO THE SUBCONSCIOUS

The hereditary principle would obviously be accepted by the neurologists, or those of them, like Critchley, who support the concept of a congenitally-determined specific dyslexia (and other reading disabilities which may or may not be of hereditary origin). It would also be acceptable to other "physical" theorists of various schools of thinking who might subscribe to the importance of symptomatology of physical defects, some of which might be hereditary in particular cases. For these might be demonstrated to their satisfaction as having been frequently concomitant with the occurrence of reading problems in the family concerned, or suspected at least of determining the occurrence of such a problem in a particular individual.

Also, the importance of heredity would be allowed by the psychoanalytically-oriented school of psychologists and psychiatrists, *not as absolute determiner* of the occurrence of reading disability in a given instance, but as a possible *pre-disposing* factor in some cases. In other words where a child with one kind of heredity —physical or otherwise—might be prone to pass through an unfavourable "climate" at critical points in the course of his psychosexual development, especially the early months, another child might be less prone to such a reaction.

In this chapter we shall look at what some of the psychoanalysts have to say, and in the next chapter, the neurologists.

Some Unconscious Factors in Reading

With this as the title of his paper, James Strachey (1930) has the following to say about printed matter and its symbolism—as seen by (some) of the psychoanalysts:

According to Freud, the book stands for a woman, and it will now be seen that this by no means contradicts Ernest Jones's interpretation of printed matter as faeces. For if the book symbolizes the mother, its author must be the father; and the printed words, the author's thoughts, fertilizing and precious, yet defiling the virgin page, must be the father's penis or faeces within the mother. And now comes the reader, the son, hungry, voracious and defiling in his turn, eager to force his way into his mother, to find out what is inside her, to tear his father's traces out of her, to devour them, to make them his own, and to be fertilized by them himself.

And so Freud is interpreted, and his thinking expounded, added to the thinking of others, re-interpreted, re-expounded, and so on ad infinitum.

It is my belief that the psychoanalysts have not succeeded in establishing the symbolism of printed matter . . . that is, that printed material in itself has special significance. Some dyslexics use printed texts to good effect in mathematics, and it is hard to see how this could be so if repressed impulses—aggression, feelings of guilt, and the like—lay behind innocent-looking shapes and combinations of symbols.

Nevertheless, Strachey's quotation has been included, not only because it is interesting, but also, because to some extent, it states an opinion which, in general terms, would be held by the psychoanalytic writers whose cases are reported in the next section of this Chapter, and in Chapter 6. In other words, these writers would claim that printed matter has symbolic significance, although without doubt they would differ at times as to the interpretation of that significance. I am of the opinion, however, that the tension relief and consequent reading improvement reported in connection with these cases was the outcome of a good psycho-therapeutic relationship established with the patients and that the success achieved did not depend on the theoretical validity of the claim regarding symbolism, or even of the total concept of psychoanalysis itself.

Phyllis Blanchard

Among the famous names that have been associated with the Philadelphia Child Guidance Clinic is that of Phyllis Blanchard, whose thinking was along psychoanalytic lines, and whose interests included problems of reading. Although her papers go back to the 'forties (some earlier) many are relevant to psychoanalytic thought on the topic of reading, today.

Blanchard divides reading disabilities into two categories: disabilities of neurotic origin and disabilities of non-neurotic origin.

The distinction she makes is: With the non-neurotic group, emotional conflicts or disturbances have arisen, in the main, out of the situation of failure in learning to read—a situation which in itself is upsetting to the child, and which is further complicated by the child's reaction to the attitude of parents and teachers to the problem. With the neurotic group, on the other hand, emotional and personality difficulties have preceded the development of the reading disability; so that the reading disability in this group is a neurotic symptom that has grown from the earlier maladjustments.

Blanchard, like Gates (1941), believes that about 75 per cent of problem readers show signs of emotional and personality disturbance, in most of whom (about three-quarters) the emotional problem is caused by the reading problem, but in one-quarter of whom the reading problem is caused by or arises out of the emotional problem.

Blanchard reviews the historical approach in the 1920s and 1930s; she herself (1946) postulates "a common ætiological factor", namely "difficulty in handling aggression, with excessive guilt and anxiety over hostile, destructive, or sadistic impulses and phantasies, which frequently were oral in form".

She sees at least some reading problems as a means of relief of anxiety and guilt about repressed instinctive drives. The relief would be by way of "the self-punishment of illness or securing punishment from others".

It was the opinion of Anna Freud (and others) that aggressive drives (against animals and people) may be sublimated by turning their energy into constructive rather than destructive activities and into the accomplishment of all kinds of tasks. By school entry time a start may be made at least in the sublimation of sexual interest and aggression.

However, a child who has not by then acquired much capacity for sublimation, may be unable to seize the opportunity for it afforded by the learning situation. In this way he may become a poor student in all subjects, and a behaviour problem as well.

Blanchard sees these mechanisms at work in reading problems also, but based on severe unconscious conflicts; the outcome is depletion of the child's energy in maintaining repression, with insufficient left over to carry through a complex mental process such as learning to read.

Moreover, this type of child often tends to resort to restriction of ego activities in order to escape painful situations and may now utilize this defence mechanism to avoid the painful experience of seeing classmates excel his achievement.

So he avoids competition, even in reading.

The plausability of this relatively mild exposition of psycho-analytic theorising makes it interesting and tempting, but one has the feeling always that "proof" is lacking—and indeed it is.

In line with the best practice in psychotherapy and psychiatry (but all too frequently lacking) the need for help to the parent is stressed where the child's problem resides at least in part in chronic child-home situations. In other words, there is need to "alter" the environment as well as the child, if maximum benefit is to accrue.

Apart from the mechanics of reading—which in the primary grades may necessitate a quite complicated "mental process", there is the problem, according to the psychoanalysts, of the *symbolism* which we have referred to briefly already, and which the child may find hard to bear. Content, too, may give rise to its own problems, for the content of the material being read becomes associated with "emotional conflicts"—certain words or combinations of words or letters and combinations of letters.

CASE STUDIES

As instances of what Blanchard has in mind, she quotes (1946) a number of cases that came her way at the clinic:

Case 1: Concerns a twelve-year-old boy, Matthew, of high I.Q. (133), whose father was in and out of work and displaced anxiety about himself and his employment difficulties from himself to excessive worry about his son's future, placing great emphasis on school success as a preparation for success in a career. The father began to supervise the boy's school work from third grade, and although the boy received good marks in reading from his teachers, his father was of the opinion that he was well below standard in this subject, and began tutoring him in it. Both the parent and the boy became upset during these lessons, and progress in reading at school slowed down, so that when Matthew reached fifth grade he was still at third-grade level in reading. He had become very sensitive to criticism about his work from teachers and was ready to fight any fellow pupil who teased him.

The therapist was unable to induce the parent to cease tutoring the boy at home. A solution was found by sending him to boarding school, where he received trained remedial teaching and learned to read satisfactorily.

Case 2: Patrick—a boy of normal intelligence (I.Q. 105), 9 years old, but could not read, despite remedial teaching provided at school. There had been three children in the family—an elder brother who had died, and a younger sister.

Anyone who deals with reading problem cases, especially if it involves detailed parental interviews, as is the case with the author, soon becomes aware of a frequently appearing source of neurotic conflicts and reading trouble—unfavourable comparison with another child, brother or sister, in the family circle. Phrases such as "she's a different child altogether", "reads like the wind", etc., betray the difficult home problem the client has, with unfavourable comparisons of this kind. In Patrick's case, however, the unfavourable comparison which caused the reading problem was between a living child and a dead brother, and Patrick was able after a time to put this into words himself.

Before looking more closely at Patrick's case, I must hasten to allay the guilt feelings of anyone who reads the preceding paragraph, is a parent and sees it as applying to him, when it may not do so. I have in mind numerous instances of family groups where a child—perhaps one of the younger ones—is so quick and able at whatever he attempts that it would be impossible to disguise the difference in potential between him and one or more other members of the family. Some parents have bent over backwards, diligently trying to help the less able child by over-compensation to the point where instead of relieving the problem, it is intensified.

Back to Patrick. He told the therapist that his brother had died just a little before he himself commenced in first grade. He explained that he had been given a book as a birthday gift about a year later, but he did not like it; the stories (which were read to him) were about people who had been killed and this upset him, so much so that he developed a strong aversion to books, never wanted to have a book read to him again, or to read a book himself.

In the early interviews with the therapist he made a strong point of love for his mother and for his dead brother, and stressed his wish always to be kind and good to people. It was apparent, however, that he was becoming jealous of other patients at the clinic, and was angry with the therapist for seeing them. He soon put this into words, maintaining that the therapist was just like his teachers, preferring other children to him.

After a time his complaints increased; the mother for whom he had professed such love was now accused of never really having loved him, but of having loved the dead brother. He told the therapist that his mother often talked about his dead brother, telling Patrick that, unlike himself, the brother had learned to read quickly and criticising Patrick for his disability.

"I wouldn't want to be like my brother," Patrick asserted. "Maybe he could read but he couldn't stand up for himself with the other kids. I'm a good fighter. They don't pick on me."

Patrick's hitherto hidden aggression against his brother now rapidly came more and more into the open. He said his mother visited the grave each week and shed tears when she was there. His previously expressed wishes to be good and kind were thrown aside. He said that he would like to dig up his brother's body and bury it somewhere so far away that his mother would never succeed in finding it; better still, he would like to burn the body and get rid of it once and for all. He said that he hated his mother when he believed that she would rather that his brother had lived and he had died, and he hated the therapist and his teachers when they seemed to prefer other children to him.

This is not a case of advancement to a happy solution, because the mother was unco-operative with the clinic. She had come along in the first place only because the school had pressed her to do so, and mostly failed to keep her appointments with the social worker, sending the boy along by himself for interviews with the therapist. After a time she withdrew him altogether, before his programme of assistance had gone far enough. But the case is interesting as an illustration of what might be behind the manifestation of a reading problem and the ætiology of the boy's disability.

When he first came to the clinic his conflicts about his mother and brother were unconscious and his hostility and resentment had been repressed. He erected for himself defence mechanisms to enable him to maintain the repression; these mechanisms were his frequently expressed wishes to be kind and good.

Blanchard interprets the development of Patrick's reading disability, as follows:

The book with stories about people being killed naturally stirred up the repressed aggressive drives and threatened to bring them into his conscious experience. In turn, this aroused feelings of guilt and anxiety (he wept whenever he saw the book) . . . as he came closer to awareness of his hostility towards his mother and his dead brother. Thus another defence and way of maintaining the repressions was refusal to learn to read, for he feared that reading content might release aggressive impulses. Self-assertion through being different from his brother was indicated by his stating his preference for being a good fighter rather than a good reader and his desire not to be like his brother. This was another motive influencing his negative attitude towards reading. Again, not learning to read was a disguised expression of hostility toward the mother who wanted him to be clever in this respect.

Case 3: A case illustrating how an event may re-activate the unconscious feelings that accompanied an earlier event of a traumatic nature:

Thomas—an eleven-year-old with an estimated I.Q. of 108 (may have been higher) and failing fifth grade for the second time. His school work was handicapped by reading disability, and he stated that the disability had begun early in third grade when a teacher of whom he was very fond had to enter hospital for an operation. She did not return to the school and the boy feared that she had died. He told the therapist that he worried so much over the teacher that he was unable to attend properly to his school work and his reading in particular soon fell behind.

A history of the boy's earlier years revealed that when he was five years old his mother had had to have an operation in hospital: but Thomas did not recall any of this or how he felt at the time; all he was able to remember was his anxiety at the absence of the teacher.

During some of the interviews Thomas asked permission to read aloud. It quickly became apparent when he did so, that every now and again the content of what he was reading would bring up unconscious emotional conflicts. He would be going along quite well, when suddenly he would make many errors, and could not continue without stopping and talking of personal matters which had been suggested to him by something he had just read.

An illustration of this was the occasion when he was reading a story about a dog. He began making the usual errors; he paused and told the therapist of a dog he once had which he loved very much, but which he was not permitted to keep. When his dog had been given away, he became very lonely, crying a great deal and wondering if it was all right. He said: "I was afraid my dog might die without my knowing about it; it is awful to be wondering whether someone you love is alive or dead".

Therapy did move on to a desirable conclusion in this case; he was able to read, after a time, without breaking down and school progress in general became satisfactory.

Case 4: This is an instance of the immediate effect of an emotionally traumatic experience in the life of a child who was separated from her mother at the time when she entered school.

Ethel was placed in a boarding school just before she turned six. This was necessary because her mother was a widow—the father had died two years previously and the mother had to go out to work. The school at once had a problem persuading Ethel to eat, but when the mother came on visits and brought food with her, the little girl ate heartily and willingly.

Along with the eating problem there ran a further one—she had great difficulty with her reading lessons, and indeed at the end of two years in the school was virtually unable to read at all. At this point (8 years of age) she was brought along for clinical help.

During the first interview the therapist formed the opinion that both the refusal to eat and the reading failure were symptoms of her emotional problems arising from the separation from her mother. While this is a fairly obvious conclusion to draw, her behaviour in play therapy both bears this out and is interesting in itself. She had spoken of her love for her mother, but attitudes of anger and hostility were soon dramatized in her play with dolls. The little girl doll, angry with the mother doll, prevented the mother from having anything to eat in the hope that she would starve her to death, and this would be just punishment for sending the little girl doll away to school. But this "bad" treatment of the mother brought punishment to the girl doll, and the girl doll "felt" ill and weak and could not eat.

Further, the little girl doll refused to read—or to study—at school. The school (in the dramatic play situation) sent reports of poor work home to the mother doll, who decided that the school was unsatisfactory *and took the baby doll home with her.*

Once she had worked her way through play with the dolls, Ethel was able to talk about her feelings when first she was sent to boarding school and could see the parallel between what was going on in her own life and what happened with the dolls. But, with new insight, Ethel saw and accepted the reality of the situation; no real home to go back to, her father dead and her mother working to support herself and the girl. She felt sympathetic to her mother and was aware that the non-eating, non-reading problem at school was adding further worries to her mother who, however, would still be unable to take her away. With insight came relief; she announced her intention to eat and sought help in her reading problem. Her symptoms disappeared and her school progress became normal.

The treatment in these cases varied: some mainly therapeutic, with little or no remedial teaching, but in this case (when the time was ripe) remedial reading helped as well.

Sometimes the remedial help is itself the general therapy for the child, having beneficial results beyond the immediate reading improvement situation. A parent will say to us: "If there had been *no* improvement in reading, the change in attitude and application and general personality change would have warranted enrolment in the reading programme."

The cases instanced by Blanchard (and there are others which time and space will not permit us to discuss) have been included as the best means of illustrating the thinking that lies behind the psycho-analytic approach to the problem of reading. That some children have to cope with a great burden of emotional disturbance at the beginning (and later) school years is certain; but it must be remembered that unwilling placement in boarding schools, outright rejection by one or both parents, cruelty, deprivation of one kind or another, death of a parent, separation and divorce, are not the only precursors to breakdown, or the "occasions" for earlier, more deep-seated conflicts to manifest themselves, as reading or other disabilities—subtler, and just as keenly felt problems in the home or school may suffice for this purpose. And it is the child living in the more subtly disturbing environment that one sees most frequently in a reading clinic.

One of the more spectacular cases involved a boy of eight years, born illegitimately to a woman with another illegitimate child. When the mother married the father of the latter child and placed the boy with an agency, ultimately deserting him completely, not only did he develop a reading disability of a marked kind and aggressive attitudes at first symbolically expressed, later more openly, but he was able to give his own version of why he used reversals in words and phrases (mirror writing): he was Jewish, his mother was not, so therefore by writing from right to left as the Hebrews do he could avoid the writing methods of the mother he (by now) said he hated. Interspersed with aggressive, "hatred" action, went periods of phantasy when he saw himself as a baby, living with his mother and cared for tenderly by her; she even (in the phantasy) cleaned up the mess caused by his enuresis.

Not all psychoanalysts would view these cases as Bdanchard does, for, as suggested earlier, there are shades of opinion amongst psychoanalysts, both as to theory and practice, and these divisions are increasing. For example, Anna Freud and Melanie Klein, two of the best known names in psycho-analysis, differ sharply in theory and in treatment of children. Anna Freud maintains that it is important to establish good relations with the young patient, but not to interpret (to the child) the material that comes up in analysis—at least not until the analysis has been going on for a considerable time. She stresses mainly the need for a friendly, supportive approach to the patient. Melanie Klein, on the other hand, is not concerned with the establishment of a "therapeutic alliance" as such, and insists that immediate interpretation of material in the analysis should be made to the child, as would be done with an adult.

To a certain extent, the clinical help is seen by some present day psychoanalysts as coming through an improvement in "object relations", rather than with a primary concern for the unravelling of an oedipus (boy-mother), or elektra (girl-father) situation. Indeed, some would go so far, I believe, as to say that the *content* of the unconscious is no longer the main concern in "transference",[4] by the analyst. One feels at times, when reading cases of interpretations and partial re-formulations of theory in some current analytic writings, that if the newer emphases are correct, Freud must surely have been unaware of certain implications of his original theorizing!

However, by whatever means the approach is made, the analysis of the infantile situation in the life of a patient would probably still be the goal of treatment.

A further discussion of psychoanalytic opinion, with further cases described, will be found later in this book (Chapter 6).

---

[4] The relationship with the analyst which involves transferring by the patient of certain feelings and impulses of aggression and love, to the analyst.

4

THE SLOW DEVELOPMENT THEORY

A Word from the Neurologists

I opened this book with a reference to a medical report of 1896 by Dr Pringle Morgan. Other medical practitioners both in general practice and in specialities such as neurology, psychiatry and opthalmology, have displayed interest and sometimes research activity into this strange phenomenon of inability to read in a person who appears to lack any physiological or anatomical impairment or dysfunction. In this chapter we shall consider the views put forward by some of the neurologists, especially Macdonald Critchley, Consulting Neurologist at King's College Hospital, London, and Consulting Physician, National Hospital, Queen Square, London.

The interest of the medical profession in this problem has been continuous since the turn of the century at least. Additional to Pringle Morgan other names come at once to mind, such as those of James Hinshelwood (a Glasgow eye-surgeon whose note to *The Lancet* on the topic of visual memory and word-blindness prompted Morgan to write to the Medical Journal about the case we have noted); Dr James Kerr, Medical Health Officer of Bradford, England (reported by Critchley, 1964); Dr Samuel T. Orton (1931, 1937), of the Greene County Mental Clinic, in Iowa; Knud Hermann (1959), a neurologist at University Hospital, Copenhagen, and many others far too numerous to mention.

Critchley's contributions to the discussions on this topic may be consulted in detail in his monograph, "Developmental Dyslexia" (1964), and various published papers, especially the William Copeland Memorial Lecture delivered at the Children's Hospital, Washington, D.C., in March, 1966. Therefore only the highlights of his hypothesis need be mentioned here. It is important however that reference to the opinions of a well-known neurologist should be included in this book, along with those of other major disciplines or schools of thought. This applies especially to Critchley as the newspapers have published several articles based on his monograph, and a notion has been growing among parents that "someone" has said that dyslexics are born, not made, and this probably fits the picture with one (or more) of their children whose reading has been a problem.

There was a period in fact (fairly recently) when it was not uncommon for a mother to announce on arrival at the clinic that her child is a dyslexic and she understands that this is an inborn difficulty in the nervous system, so she supposes there is not much that can be done about it—or will ask anxiously, "Do you think he is a dyslexic?" The word had a good sound to it, and if your child "had" it, it was a good topic of conversation; if it was mysteriously rooted in the "nervous system", it was worth talking about even more. We have already noted how this kind of thinking crept into the description of her son given to me recently by a woman medical practitioner.

Specific Disability

Critchley is careful (as was Hallgren) to distinguish in his thinking between the syndrome of congenital dyslexia (developmental dyslexia, specific dyslexia, or call it what you will) and other cases of reading disability. Whether he has succeeded, however, where I feel so many others have failed, namely, in clearly establishing not only the theoretical possibility of such an entity, but the feasibility of detecting it in the diagnosis of a particular case, is another matter.

He puts it in these words (1964):

When neurologists demarcated "congenital word blindness" as an entity, they did not for a moment intend to embrace the whole community of illiterates, semi-illiterates, poor readers, slow readers, retarded readers, bad spellers, or reluctant writers.

He also takes to task the members of other disciplines—pedagogy and psychology—which have "assumed a more active and even aggressive role". He denies that the various forms of reading disability can be regarded as parts of a continuum—"something which ranged from intellectual inadequacy at one end of the scale, to neurosis at the other".

Critchley is not denying the fact that emotional disturbance is observable in many cases of reading disability, but he takes a very different view of that from psychoanalysts, for instance, or psychologists, who (he says) in speculating about these emotional symptoms, have permitted the blame for the reading problem to fall on "one scapegoat after another, the teacher, the parents and the child".

Fortunately, the psychologists and educators are not the only ones taken to task. "Even among medical writers there has also been some confused thinking on occasions." And in this connection he cites (1966) arguments put forward at times concerning birth trauma and dyslexia, or the possibility of dyslexia's occurring more frequently where the mother has had many children.

In an essay to the Royal Statistical Society in 1896, Dr James Kerr had referred to "a boy who can do arithmetic well so long as it involves Arabic numerals only, but writes gibberish in a neat hand for dictation exercise".

This tendency to obsessiveness and perseverativeness in some severe reading cases is apparent to those who have anything to do with them. A particularly severe case referred to the writer by a psychiatrist, and until recently in the clinic, meticulously copies down whatever he is set to, dotting the "i's" and crossing the "t's", and with a neat hand like the Kerr case (many, of course, are very poor writers, often illegible); another boy who comes to mind will not make a move with a task until he has written in the exact heading, underlined it, added any other marks—such as page numbering—that are customary with him and cannot be persuaded to start until he has done so.

Late Developers

By the term "developmental dyslexia", Critchley refers to the concept held by men like Apert (1924) and Pötzl (1924) of a delay in development—a "maturational lag"—so that dyslexics would be slow developers (as far as reading is concerned), "late bloomers", as he says, "to use that faintly ridiculous term". The idea of some structural brain defect will not hold water, and in the Copeland lecture (1966) he answers his rhetorical question, "Is developmental dyslexia the expression of minor cerebral damage?" with an expected and emphatic "no".

Acceptance by the neurologists of the hereditary concept would render any theory supporting the idea of birth injury as a cause of developmental dyslexia at least improbable, from their point of view. But this does not rule out severe birth injury and other brain damage as the possible cause of some reading problems.

A summary of the clinical assessment a neurologist might make of the dyslexic would be one disclosing no history of problems in the mother during pregnancy, the child being born at term, normal in weight, ordinarily of healthy appearance, "without trace of neonatal jaundice, or of cyanosis, and no digestive or elimination difficulties". "The first twelve months," says Critchley, "are generally uneventful. The infant cuts its first teeth at the expected age, and holds up its head, sits, stands and walks according to the normal scale." It is sometimes alleged that some of the children later diagnosed by neurologists as dyslexics omit the crawling stage, but the question arises—what proportion of "normal" children also omit this stage? There may be little, if any, difference. One fact, however, is supported by all known authorities and cannot be gainsaid—the number of boys with reading problems is much greater than the number of girls. This may be partly due to sociological or domestic reasons—a reading disability may attract more attention and concern in a boy than it would in a girl, but this is unlikely to be the whole story.

Some neurologists who deal mainly with children are of the opinion that a statistically significant number of dyslexics are slow in learning to talk, while some give evidence of dyslalia (imperfect speech) and are in need of speech therapy. This is not universally accepted, but would merit further study.

The medical-neurological examination of a dyslexic does not uncover any striking abnormality, in general, or of the nervous system in particular. Critchley instances lack of traces of spasticity, while vision and hearing tests are satisfactory.

Dominance and Laterality

The problem of cerebral dominance is naturally of interest to a neurologist, but it is pointed out that not many dyslexics are found to possess firm dominance—left or right—as regards brain function, and many appear to be crossed laterals, although the determination of left- or right-handedness, -footedness and -eyedness is not a simple matter. Also among the non-dyslexics, many cases of crossed dominance and of sinistrality or left-handedness, -footedness, etc., are found.

It must be admitted that the notion of dominance and laterality as an important ætiological factor in reading disability has been discarded by many theorists, but the clinician with his day-to-day

cases of reading problems (not just the "pure" dyslexics) is frequently struck with the number of pencils held in left hands that
he sees in a day. The feeling is that there may very well be some
link here.

Critchley feels that mixed laterality, or sidedness with no clear-
cut cerebral dominance, may prove to be a more significant
ætiological factor in dyslexia than sinistrality has proven to be.
He also feels that the claim put forward by some writers that the
dyslexic often displays clumsiness—of gait, of manual dexterity,
and so on—must be treated with caution. What is the definition of
clumsiness, and how do we measure it? Indeed, where an alleged
dyslexic does display unusual awkwardness, the monograph suggests that the possibility must be seriously considered that the
difficulty in reading in such a case is perhaps "an epiphenomenon
of serious brain damage".[5]

Investigation of Spacial Concepts and Manipulations

"Potential" dyslexics, it is sometimes suggested, are late in
learning to tell the time and their drawings may be unusual—a
bicycle may be drawn in parts, instead of the whole thing, points
of the compass drawn on a map or plan may be confused, certain
letters (b, d, etc.) may be disoriented both when the child writes
a word or manipulates cardboard or plastic letters. There would
not be general agreement, however, as to the value of these as
early pointers to the possibility of development of dyslexia in a
child, or even that they are pointers at all (author's comment).

Critchley summarizes, in the Copeland lecture, an important
component of the extended neurological examination of the alleged
dyslexic, namely that of the child's concept of sidedness. The
patient is asked to indicate his right hand, right foot, ear, eye, etc.,
and then to "cross-over", touching the right ear with the left hand,
and so on. Next he is asked to indicate the examiner's right hand,
or left hand (or foot), then to indicate which is the right object
and which is the left object in groups of inanimate paired objects
such as gloves or shoes. Finally there are tests that he says often
seem hardest of all—to indicate the right or left side of a doll
which is held up, both facing the child, and with its back to the
child.

Schilder and Hoff have described abnormal postures of the
upper limbs brought about by passively moving the head and neck

---

[5] Or is this just a way of saying, "dyslexics, in diagnostic examination, do
not dislpay unusual awkwardness, but if they do they are not dyslexics"?

—postures which, they claim, disappear in normal children at about seven years of age, but may continue in dyslexics for another five years or so. It is stated that this is true also of the phenomenon of ability to maintain accurately an attitude of the outstretched arms by a patient who has his eyelids closed.

In describing these symptoms, Critchley is insistent that diagnosis of dyslexia must be made by a neurologist, and if he and his fellows are correct in their claim that there is a specific dyslexia of neurological origin, they are right in doing so, at least as far as that particular abnormality is concerned. It is not necessary, therefore, to add a more detailed description of neurological signs to look for in examination, although quite a few of those listed above could be detected by any intelligent examiner, no matter what his training.

There has been some report of records of eye movements of dyslexics while attempting to read, which are said to be (as one would expect) very erratic. This is interesting to me as I have had considerable experience in photographing the reading movements of people's eyes (mostly children) by means of a reading-eye camera or opthalmograph. This is never easy, even with a "normal" reader and always difficult to obtain with a problem reader, if for no other reason than the fact that such a person cannot read the card well enough to have his eye movements photographed.

How one could photograph the reading eye movements of a child or adult with a reading problem sufficient to have him labelled "dyslexic" by the neurologists, it is hard to imagine. The eye-movement "traces" of, say, poor readers whose problem is known to have onset following some traumatic experience (physical or emotional), are very erratic. Is it being said that the developmental dyslexic, if there is such a person, manifests a specific kind of erratic trace? We are not told.

I am also interested in another opinion in the monograph that "few dyslexics exhibit any defect in the realm of spoken language". The authority for this assumption is not given—it may be an impression Critchley gained in the course of clinical diagnosis, and this he is entitled to do. He also asserts that they usually have command of vocabulary similar to that of other children of their age.

Both of these claims are contrary to findings of a number of researchers (for example, Bannatyne, 1966), and to some extent of the author's own experience. Parents will sometimes tell me that the child seems to have a speech difficulty and ask me to bear it in mind during the diagnostic appraisal session, and the school reports may refer to this. It is not, however, so prominent a feature of reading disability cases seen in a clinic that it makes too strong an impression on one's mind. Without a careful appraisal and count in a large number of cases (which I have not so far done), what statistical significance (if any) this symptom, or alleged symptom, might prove to have, I do not know.

There are, however, among the severe cases that are at the same time the most severe emotional cases—such as those referred by psychiatrists—I believe a greater percentage of speech disabilities. With children of this kind, the speech sometimes seems to follow somewhat tortuous paths, to some extent reminiscent of the reading —as though the problem is not one of organ defect of tongue, larynx, etc., but something of a more central nature, with the child groping for the pronunciation of a word, in the same way that his eye gropes for recognition of the visual symbol; and this "groping" may be noticed in *talking* with the clinician, apart from reading aloud (where one would expect to find speech hesitancies, strange word forms and so on).

May Be Wrongly Classified

In cases especially where there are fairly severe emotional and/or anti-social tendencies partly due to the sense of frustration and "difference" often felt by very poor readers, a child may be at first neglected in a large class, and later segregated as a suspected case of poor ability, or even as a delinquent. Some children in "secondary activity" classes are later found to have good ability, admission to the classes having been "gained" in the manner suggested above. There may not be many instances of unfortunate classification and segregation of this kind but, to the author's knowledge, there are undoubtedly more than there should be.

Hinshelwood (1902), the Glasgow eye surgeon already referred to, put it like this:

It is a matter of highest importance to recognise the cause and true nature of this difficulty in learning to read, which is experienced by these children, otherwise they may be harshly neglected or punished.

If dyslexia is a neurological entity and has to do with the written word as such—not merely the adequacies or inadequacies of the spelling system used—one would expect to find poor readers in more or less phonetic language countries such as Germany, Czechoslovakia and Italy, and this is in fact the case.

This certainly must be an arresting thought to those who, from time to time, have alleged that the inconsistent spelling in English-speaking countries is an important factor in reading disability in those countries. But that is a long way from claiming that this substantially supports the view of the existence of a specific dyslexia of neurological origin, with which a person may be born.

Critchley's monograph and other writings have undoubtedly made a very important contribution to current thinking about severe reading problems. Unfortunately (as I see it), the stand taken by him is absolute and unequivocal. There are few if any "ifs" and "buts", and this gives his arguments an authoritative standing with many people, but it is disquieting to those of us who see difficulties in diagnosis no matter who carries out the task, and prefer to take a broader view.

He writes (1964):

Some educationalists have surely been both muddled and opiniated upon this problem . . . Neurologists too have been at fault—not so much in taking up too naive a standpoint as in being reluctant to press their views sufficiently.

Named by him are some of the well-known "giants" in this field —psychologists and educational psychologists—Burt, Schonell, Vernon and Monroe.

The neurological hypothesis put forward in the monograph is that developmental dyslexia is an entity, different from other forms or instances of reading disability, but the insistence on the accuracy of the hypothesis makes one pause and question at times the case that is being made out. One feels particularly uneasy in this regard when instances that appear exactly like reported cases of developmental dyslexia, but are known to include factors (such as minor brain damage) rejected by neurologists as ætiological factors in developmental dyslexia, are set aside with the simple (but firm) statement: this case is not developmental dyslexia although it appears to be so; it is the result of brain damage (or something else) and so is not congenitally determined, whereas developmental dyslexia *is* congenitally determined.

In stressing the *developmental* aspect of the entity they have in mind, the neurologists place emphasis on the factor of immaturity with cortical developmental and processes of learning out of step with (or lagging behind) chronological age.

The trouble is, *has* the hypothesis of *maturational lag,* with immaturity in the relevant nervous or cortical development been clearly established? To the author it seems that this has not been done and, if so, the "entity" theory remains unproven.

Knud Hermann

The neurologists do not always agree among themselves, of course, any more than any other group. Thus, Knud Hermann, Chief Physician at the Neurological Unit of University Hospital, Copenhagen, refers (1959) to a syndrome '"Gerstmann's Syndrome"), which, he says, presents a picture something like that of developmental dyslexia, but which is not always due to constitutional or inherited factors. It is also called the parietal syndrome, because it is said to be due to disease of a circumscribed area of the parietal lobe. However, the existence of this syndrome as a specific entity is by no means universally accepted by his colleagues.

Gerstmann, an Austrian neurologist, described the syndrome that bears his name, in 1924, listing as the most important symptoms:

1. Disorientation in right-left dimensions.
2. Finger agnosia.
3. Acalculia (difficulty with figures).
4. Agraphia, because of:
    (*a*) deformed letters;
    (*b*) confused letter shapes;
    (*c*) reversals.

It would appear that spelling may be satisfactory with Gerstmann's Syndrome, whereas poor spelling is almost an invariable accompaniment of severe reading disability, or even mild reading disability; and acalculia is *not* a necessary or even frequent accompaniment of reading disability, as reported in cases in the literature, or in the author's own experience. Indeed, a parent frequently says at interview: "He's all right [or she] at arithmetic", or "he does well at arithmetic or mathematics in general".

Diagnosis—A Check List

It is in the diagnosis of dyslexia that one feels most uneasy about claims that it is a congenital entity. We have seen that it is hard to pin down specific neurological or other physical signs and when lists of errors made by an allegedly dyslexic child when reading are perused, anyone working in this field realises at once that they are met with—sometimes all of them, always many of them—in any case of severe reading disability, including cases with a history of physical (brain) trauma.

Critchley,[6] in his turn, has compiled such a list, covering seventeen errors, and in brief they are set down here:

1. Wild guesses at phonetic structure of unfamiliar words.
2. Confusion in "similar" words; or reversals: PUB-BUD; ON-NO.
3. Difficulty in detecting difference in *sounds* of words or letters.
4. Frequent losing of place when reading.
5. Difficulty in sweeping eyes accurately from right end of one line to left end of next line.
6. Vocalisation—reading aloud, or almost reading aloud (subvocalisation) when one is supposedly reading silently.
7. Reading with poor or nil comprehension.
8. Vowels incorrectly pronounced (BAG-BIG), etc.
9. Consonants incorrectly pronounced (BOLD-BOLT).
10. Reversals (partly referred to in 2 above: WAS-SAW; DID HE-HE DID; or mirror-opposite letters: DIP-BID, etc.
11. Interpolation of phonemes: TRICK for TICK.
12. Omission of phonemes: TICK for TRICK; or syllable omission: WALK for WALKING.
13. Complete word substitution: WAS for LIVED.
14. Perseveration or repetition: THE CAT THE CAT THE CAT.
15. Addition of words (appropriate or otherwise): e.g., ONCE THERE WAS may be read ONCE UPON A TIME THERE WAS.
16. Omission of a complete word or words; for A FIERCE DOG reading A DOG.
17. "Refusals"—baulking at a word: thus for ONE OF THE MOST INTERESTING a child may read: ONE OF THE MOST and stop firmly at that point.

The neurologists have little to say about the influence of emotional factors—or even the presence of emotional maladjustment to any extent, and of course they would reject the claims of the psychoanalysts with their reliance on adverse environmental

---

6 Depending on both Monroe and Goldberg. But note that Monroe does not use the term dyslexia as a working term, and appears to disapprove of it. Refers instead to severe reading difficulty.

experience at critical ages. It would be interesting, however, to
have a psychoanalyst go over the check list above, especially the
items "baulking at a word", "word substitution" and "perseveration".

Fluctuations

A characteristic of many cases of reading disability is the pattern
of fluctuations that one sees. A child will often vary in performance level from test to test and perhaps from day to day. Even
in intelligence, there may be wide variations in results in the sub-
tests, and the more difficult items are not always the ones wrongly
answered. One could elaborate on this, but it suffices to mention it.
It may bring into question the concept of a Reading Age such as
Schonell employs—where the score in a test is referred to a chart
to ascertain the age level at which the child has performed in the
test. In any case one must consider not only the score obtained,
but the *manner* in which it was obtained; for example, a score of
35 may be obtained by attempting 60 and making errors in 25;
or by attempting 40 and making errors in 5. And so on.

Critchley maintains that developmental dyslexia is independent
of ocular defects. But there have been contrary reports from some
writers. Thus, to quote one example, Thomas Harrison Eames, an
opthalmic surgeon, studied 260 cases (114 of whom were reading
disability cases and 146 unselected school children) from his own
practice and at the Harvard Psychological Clinic in 1932, and
noted "the tendency for the reading disability groups to exhibit
poorer vision, greater degree of exophoria [7] in distance and near
vision, and lower ductions".[8]

There have been reports on some reduction in auditory power
(less severe however than reports such as the above concerning
visual material) with dyslexics; in our own clinic and in school
surveys we have carried out, neither deficient vision nor deficient
hearing appears to occur with greater statistical frequency among
poor readers, and this applies both to the severely retarded and
the mildly retarded readers.

Electro-Encephalography

There are reports from time to time of mild dysrhythmias, in

---

[7] Defined by Eames as: "Tendency for the eyes to deviate outward".

[8] "Extent to which antagonistic prism power may be introduced before
the eyes without dissociating the images."

reading disability cases, which are suggestive, the neurologists say, of cortical immaturity, but they are regarded as minor evidence.

Teaching The Dyslexic

We have already mentioned some aspects of attacking the problem by means of psychological therapy, or tutorial assistance, or both, and this is considered further in Chapter 6 and Chapter 7. Critchley set down a few basic guide-lines for the teaching of dyslexics, but they are reminiscent of writings by educationalists and psychologists and he agrees that they are not in a neurologist's field, and therefore should be left in the hands of those more immediately concerned with remedial reading. However, he stresses very firmly the need to replace the look-and-say method with a method of paying more attention to basic fundamentals and phonetics and to the use of aids which should be interesting, exciting and colourful. His opinion, if I am interpreting it correctly, is that the method itself is not important, providing it is intense and individual.

5

CAUSES AND TYPES OF READING DISABILITY

I have used the word reading disability in this heading to avoid confusion with the notion of specific (developmental) dyslexia in the previous chapter, put forward by the neurologists. However, as will be seen later in this section, it is hard to avoid all confusion, as some renowned writers, e.g., Professor Magdalen Vernon (1965), speak also of "specific dyslexia", but with a connotation different from that implied by Hallgren, or by Critchley, or (sometimes) from one another.

My use of the term dyslexia in this chapter will, as mentioned earlier, be synonymous with reading disability, unless otherwise stated.

There is a difference between a multi-causal approach (in the sense of several interlocking causal factors conjointly "producing" a particular kind of dyslexia) and the concept of various kinds of dyslexia resting mainly on one (or one kind of) causal factor, but with other factors slightly changing the picture in any particular case.

If we set about a consideration of causes and types of dyslexia, as Bannatyne (1966) who has attempted a diagrammatic representation of the classification of dyslexias, we may come up with quite a variety, but mostly they will re-group fairly comfortably into four main categories. Before going further, however, we should do well to remind ourselves that problems with reading and with language in general may arise from a number of causes, such as low I.Q., severe personality (neo-psychotic) maladjustment and aphasia or damage to language centres of the brain following accident.

Obviously we do not think of the mentally retarded individual as a reading disability case—his problem is otherwise, even though he may not (almost certainly cannot) read well, if at all. The same applies to the child or adult who is so poorly adjusted that he is seriously ill; this may have prevented him from learning to read or it may be hampering his attempts to read now. But again we think of him not as a reading problem case primarily, but as a personality deviation case, for instance, severely neurotic or psychotic.

The aphasic does at times closely resemble the dyslexic but mostly the destruction or modification of brain tissue is wider and affects language in general (sometimes in a bizarre way) rather than just reading. Brain lesions following physical traumata may very well provide us with a case of accident-determined dyslexia, but here the effect in brain and nerve is "narrower" than is the case with aphasia, and language is *not* severely handicapped.

Classification

The four groups with which we finally arrange our classification of causes and types of dyslexia will include *some* that have a factor of low intelligence (but not mental deficiency); *some* that rest on factors of maladjustment (but not of an excessive nature) and *some* that are post-traumatic in the physical sense. In the latter groups several clients come at once to my mind—a girl of 14 who had suffered head injuries in a fall from a cot during infancy; a boy of 12 with exceptionally bright siblings, and who himself had shown great promise intelligence-wise up to the age of three, when he was knocked down by a car, and sustained brain injury. He had to learn to walk and talk again (which he did after a time quite well), but was left with a residual reading difficulty which brought him to our clinic.

To digress for a moment—it has been my experience that children who showed promise in the early years and then were "set-back" by accident as the boy and girl above were, frequently give one the feeling that they are "limping behind themselves", as it were. They may test at 90 or 88 or 92 or so I.Q., but they don't seem to be quite like others in the non-accident group who score I.Q.s of that kind. And I have found that not only do they benefit in personality as their remedial reading progresses, but they do better in other areas of life (school and home and elsewhere) and sometimes *score significantly better* at an I.Q. re-test later.

Bannatyne, who is Director of the Word Blind Centre for Dyslexic Children, London, groups as a "sub-species" under the genera Primary Emotional Dyslexia, children whose mothers are either disinterested in them, or are severely depressed or who are continuously angry and punishing. With such mothers there must be a poor communicative relationship, resulting in slow and hesitant speech, poor vocabulary and an inability to *listen* properly or to respond effectively to auditory stimuli. With the depressed mother, for example, laughter on either side will be evoked infrequently, and a child beset by continuous haranguing from an angry mother, reinforced by slaps and beatings, develops a great deal of anxiety and words trouble him.

With the dyslexias arising from neurological dysfunction (caused by disease or accident in the main) we may have visuo-spatial disorders, auditory or hearing disorders and "integrative disorders" (where the mechanisms and nerve pathways enabling integration of stimulus input, habit formation and output channels are inefficient). There would also be the motor-kinaesthetic group where necessary muscle movement and co-ordination are lacking to a greater or lesser degree.

And, of course, combinations of these kinds of neurological disorders may be found in the same individual.

Varying Techniques

Bannatyne believes that for each type of disorder there must be an appropriate remedial technique. That children with a visuo-spatial deficiency must be trained with spatial techniques, a child with auditory discrimination disorders must be assisted with appropriate techniques to encourage careful listening and accurate speaking, while the motor-kinaesthetic child, or child also with tactile (touch) problems will require attention to these disabilities while his total reading problem is being assisted.

Having discussed in some detail the opinion of geneticists such as Hallgren (familial instances) and Critchley et al (congenital, developmental problems) we may pass over the groups labelled genetic dyslexia with little more than a mention. The concept of a "continuum" or smooth scale including us all and running from the very poor readers to the very good readers is again put forward.

One concept that is both interesting and, I think, important, is that of the "level of functioning". How many music "dyslexics" or drawing "dyslexics" would there be if we were all expected to write and understand simple symphonic music or perform satisfactorily in varying kinds of art media. I suppose it is more reasonable to expect a greater number of people to read and write sophisticated material, but to what extent should this be modified in the face of one's ceiling of intelligence? We will not enter here into considerations of the usefulness or otherwise of terms such as "general ability", etc. We are not so naive about them as we once were, but they are meaningful enough in the above context. The reader will recall the statement made at the beginning of this book, that the existence of a reading problem (certainly one that can be helped) is indicated not so much by the "level" at which the child can read, as the existence or otherwise of a gap between the level at which he reads and the level at which, from an assessment of his ability, one might expect him to be able to read.

Sex Difference

We have noted that more boys than girls have reading problems. In general, girls and women score better on tests of verbal ability, are more fluent and more expressive. The active domination of the environment is important to a man; it always has been. To be poor at spatial manipulation would have endangered not only the man, but his dependent family in the cave-man days and would have prevented the rise of civilisation later with its advances in engineering and mechanics. To sense the needs of a family, a refined emotional or feeling responsiveness was essential in the woman.

I believe that this is much oversimplified, and we can all call to mind at once many instances that run counter to it. But it is interesting and may contain a germ of truth to help explain the sex difference in reading disability.

Bannatyne deals at some length with the appreciation of spatial relationships. It will be remembered that the neurologists, or Critchley at any rate, are of the opinion that crossed laterality, mixed dominance and ambidextrality have importance in the "making" of a dyslexic, more than mere sinistrality or left-handedness, eyedness, footedness, etc. Bannatyne supports this and ties it in with the sex factor in dyslexia. Stressing the need, especially in the rugged days of old, of quick grasp of the whole field of vision by the male, ambidextrality or at any rate equal-eyedness would be a great help and have survival value for the family if the males were so endowed. But it would place at least some males at a disadvantage in carrying out an exercise such as reading where the eyes for the best effect must be capable of moving in *one* direction, mainly, in *one visual field*. There is no space here to elaborate on this, but it can be seen that lack of dominance would increase the likelihood that the mirrored image (letters) in the right visual field would be fed out instead of the "correct" ones in the left visual cortex.

The males of our species, then, according to this theory, are endowed for superior spatial ability and lowered verbal (especially reading) ability.

Not only does verbal fluency seem to require this well-established dominance, but so does the interpretation of auditory processes, such as in learning to read, where the sounds of the word (i.e., the "aural sequence of phonemes") are tied up with the visual representation of the word. Thus in T-a-b-l-e we have a specific (but arbitrary) order of sounds, and the word has a specific or near specific appearance.

Treatment

If Bannatyne's theory is valid, a "genetic dyslexic"—one whose problem lies in his genes—would require help in "(*a*) auditory sequencing, (*b*) auditory discrimination and (*c*) associating auditory symbols with sequences of visual sounds". In other words, the client would require training in *listening*. Perhaps to this might be added directional (left-to-right) training of the eyes to establish satisfactory eye muscle habits.

"The evidence to hand so far suggests that fathers in highly spatial occupations, for example, surgeons, architects, engineers, farmers, tend to have more genetically dyslexic children than do fathers in other occupations. Although the mothers and daughters in these families may be linguistically superior to the males, the difference is relative because in terms of the community as a whole the verbal talents of the women will also tend to be lower than they might be. In other words, the women in 'genetic dyslexic' families . . . will exhibit minimal symptoms. For example, their ability to learn foreign languages may be limited because of a fundamental lack of talent."

Whether "the evidence to hand so far" does suggest this is, I believe, doubtful but continued research and observation with this in mind would be worthwhile.

Social, Cultural and Educational Dyslexia

Here we have the by-product of environmental factors in home, school and the world of the child, at large. Obviously the main attack must be on the environment itself where possible, including

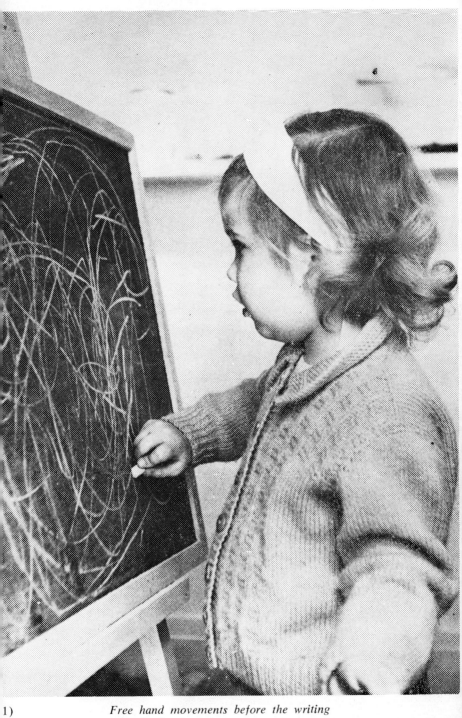

1) *Free hand movements before the writing stage begins.*

(2)

The child who can read
has an endless source
of enjoyment at hand.

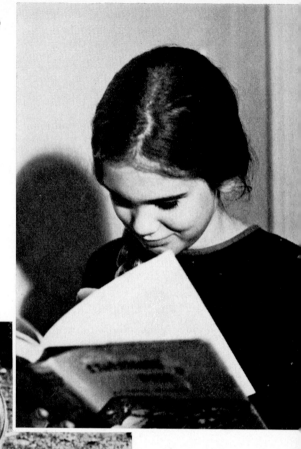

"I think I'll look at this one.

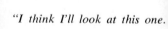

(3)

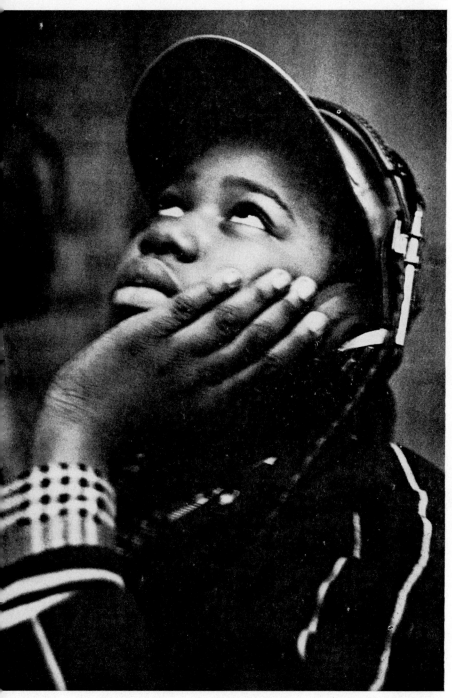

(4) *Listening skill is important to the acquisition of reading skill. This boy is in the films and recordings centre of the Cincinnati Public Library, Ohio, U.S.A.*

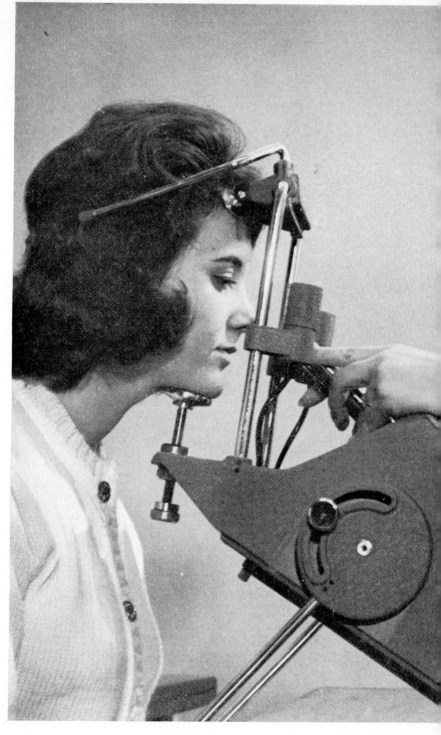

(5)

The "reading-eye" camera, or
graphing the movements of

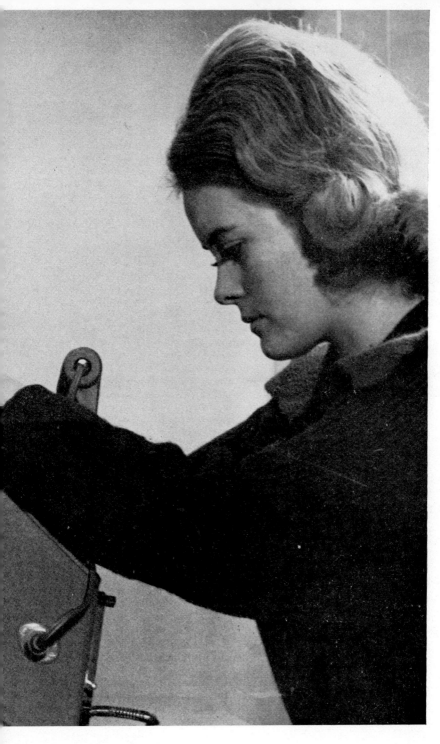

ograph — shown here photo-
of the eyes, while reading.

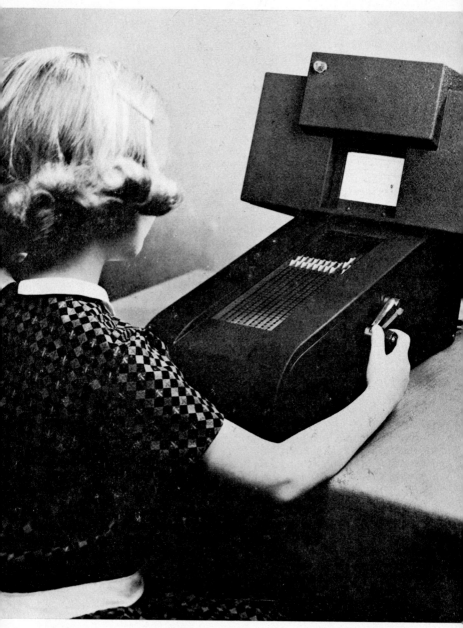

(6)   *Teaching machines, invented in the first instance by Harvard psychologist, Professor B. F. Skinner, have not yet played a major role in beginning reading or remedial reading, but there are programmes for spelling (and some for reading) and more will follow.*

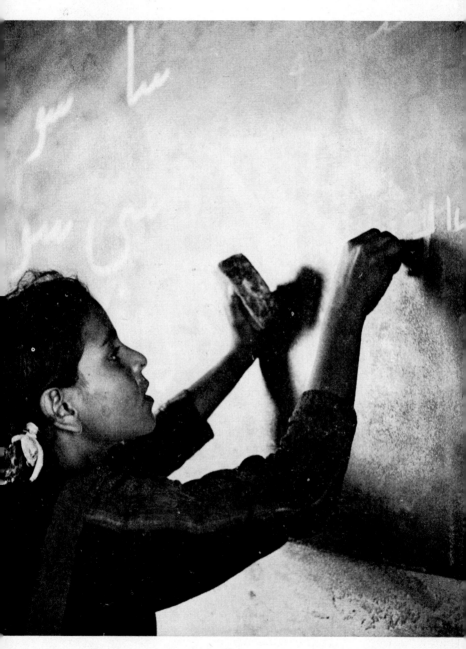

(7)   *An Arab refugee in the Gazza Strip battles with the problems of beginning Arabic writing. To a dyslexic, the printed word in English is as devoid of meaning as these Arabic symbols are to most of us.*

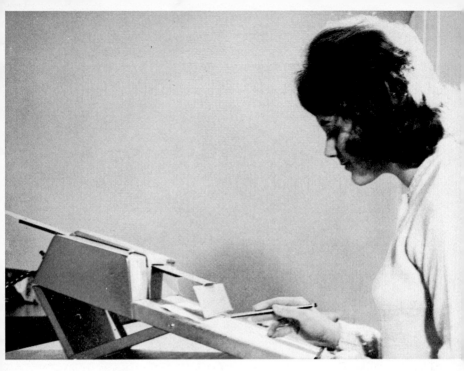

(8) *THE "READING RATE CONTROLLER".*
This type permits an individual to adjust to his own needs and speeds.

(9) *THE "TELEBINOCULAR"*
Checks for visual defects and referral to an expert.

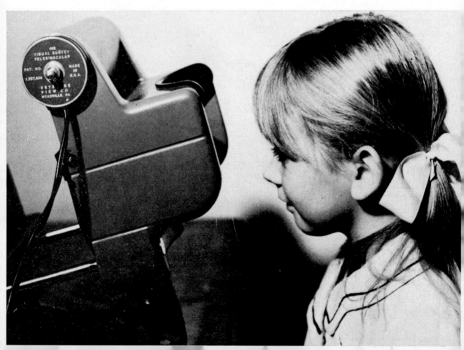

the school curriculum; for with the environment that has "caused" or made possible the dyslexia, unchanged, relief or marked improvement is unlikely. The child will need help—emotional, educational and perhaps in some cases, physical (spectacles, hearing aids, or more subtle physical assistance) concomitant with the attempt to ameliorate environmental factors, but the latter is the crux of this kind of dyslexia or reading problem.

Obviously dyslexics are not often (perhaps rarely) identifiable as belonging exclusively to one group as outlined in this chapter, but frequently the causal factors overlap. The groups are not mutually exclusive. The number of carefully standardised tests in the psychological, educational, physiological and neurological fields needed for accurate differential diagnosis would be overwhelming; but the concept of dyslexias of varying causation is useful and appears to fit the facts and to provide a helpful approach, if not pressed too far, in clinical practice. An example of "pressing it too far" would be to attempt to discover an exact cause in each case—which, by the way, many parents would like to see done. I prefer to discuss with the parent the major causal possibilities, indicating those that appear on the evidence of tests, case history and clinical observation, to be unlikely causes in a particular case, but reminding the parent that in my view and that of many others, progress can be made without an arbitrary pin-pointing of an exact cause or causes. Unhelpful environmental conditions, where these are apparent, should always be borne in mind and an attempt made to deal with them—a thing easier to do with a co-operative parent than one on the defensive, if home conditions are involved.

Professor Magdalen Vernon, who is Professor of Psychology, University of Reading, England, while supporting the multi-factorial approach to ætiology (1957, 1965), warns against rigid classification in most individual cases; she suggests three rough but possibly useful groups: (*a*) those with disorders of visual perception, (*b*) those with disorders of auditory perception, and (*c*) those who show deficiency in conceptual reasoning. She also uses the term "specific dyslexia" to include cases of severe reading disability where this is the main symptom, e.g., where major impairment in other areas is lacking. For example, she feels that where a severe emotional problem lies behind a reading problem as its probable cause, other severe problems will very likely have arisen from the same cause (that is, backwardness, apart from the backwardness arising from the reading disability itself, will tend to be more general). Here, of course, she would differ from Blanchard and others who see *some* reading disabilities of a severe nature arising from "psychological" causes with little deficiency in other learning areas.

Vernon is not entirely clear in her approach and I feel not always consistent. She supports the idea of "dyslexias" and multi-causes, but suggests also that perhaps the term dyslexia might most usefully be reserved for those cases where backwardness in reading is due to a congenital deficiency (but not in general intelligence), or to cases of minimal brain damage. Any attempt to exclude cases of maladjustment (as Vernon does)—that is, where emotional maladjustment is the primary cause of reading disability —would appear to be difficult, to say the least; *secondary* emotional causes arising with or out of the reading disability can look very like the primary maladjustment even to the experienced clinician and his tests make a poor job of sorting them out.

I prefer her statement that "there may be more than one type of dyslexia, each with its characteristic symptoms", but with over-lap, to some extent, from one kind to another; thus, as cautioned above, we should avoid over-rigid classification in any particular case. In fact, Vernon states (1957) regarding causal factors that "there is no very clear conclusive evidence that reading backward-ness is associated with any particular type of defect or emotional disorder".

At the same time, she agrees that some studies demonstrate "quite clearly that some cases of retarded reading result from emotional disorders which can be remedied by psychotherapeutic treatment". This would obviously affect only those retarded read-ers who exhibit emotional problems as well as reading difficulties, and we have already noted that there is considerable difference of opinion as to the percentage of reading cases who show signs of emotional difficulty. Thus Fernald (1943) says that only four cases out of seventy-eight extremely backward readers had any history of emotional instability prior to entering school, while Blanchard reports considerable emotional disorder in her clinic cases, and others put the figure between these two extremes. The emotionally stable backward readers would be quite unaffected in the reading proficiency by psychotherapy aimed at relieving emotional tension, for, theoretically, they are not suffering from tension.

I have given my opinion earlier, from experience with a large number of backward readers, that emotional maladjustment is *frequently* observed as a complicating factor with such children and that not only is the attention to the emotional problem likely to have a beneficial influence on the reading disability, but clinical help for the reading problem often alleviates the emotional problem and is a form of therapy for the emotional maladjustment and not merely for the reading problem.

In other words, it is possible for a clinician to say: Here we have a backward reader who is also showing signs of emotional difficulty; I do not know for sure whether (in this case) the backward reading "triggered-off" the emotional problem, or whether it is the other way round, or whether both problems have arisen from some other cause or causes (e.g., home or environmental difficulties); however, I shall regard the case mainly as an emotional maladjustment case and shall provide therapy aimed at relieving this maladjustment in the hope that not only the emotional problem, but also the reading problem will benefit as a result; (or he might decide) I shall regard the case primarily as a reading retardation case and my main concern will be to provide a suitable remedial programme, but I shall bear in mind that there is also evidence of emotional maladjustment and hope that this will be afforded some relief as the reading difficulty clears up; or he might combine the two lines of thinking and say, although I consider this case to be primarily an emotional maladjustment case, I shall provide a reading programme in the belief that this will be a suitable means of providing therapy for the emotional problem.

It must be again stressed that it is not very fruitful and may be misleading to attempt to pin down a particular circumstance or set of circumstances as *the* cause of a reading disability case, and I think that Vernon's quotation (1957) from Stewart illustrates this.

Stewart studied thirty children aged $8\frac{1}{2}$ to $12\frac{1}{2}$ years who were suffering a considerable degree of maladjustment. Half this group were superior and half were inferior readers. He found as follows:

Both sets of children were basically insecure. But the superior readers had parents who were of the rejecting type, and the children struggled to excel in reading apparently in order to win their parents' approval. They also found that reading afforded them a refuge in a world of phantasy, and a compensation for their other difficulties. The inferior readers, on the other hand, did not strive for success in reading, and had no fear of the consequences of failure, either because their parents placed no value on reading; or as an act of hostility towards their parents (the children were often of an aggressive type); or as a means of gaining the support of indulgent, over-protective or capricious parents. These findings suggest that fundamentally maladjusted children may exhibit reading backwardness as one symptom of the disorder in appropriate circumstances, possibly without any essential cognitive difficulty in learning to read.

I am glad that Vernon reminds us (1957) that others, e.g. Hattwick and Stowell in 1936 and Kent in 1955, do not corroborate these findings. However, Hattwick and Stowell do seem to have shown that "both over-protectiveness and excessive pressure exerted by parents may make it harder for children to settle down to normal school work, and hence to learn to read easily."

There is no doubt that parent-child relationships are important to success in learning to read, or, often, in failure to do so. Our own files show numerous cases of over-protectiveness and excessive pressure, but they also show that what is a suitable parent-child relationship to one child may be anything but suitable to another. Any clinical psychologist or psychiatrist is aware that one child may be distressed if a mother and father raise their eyebrows at one another at the breakfast table, while another may be secure and apparently free from stress in a home where alcoholism, continuous quarrelling, or even prostitution is present.

What is one child's meat may be another's poison.

As Vernon is certainly one of the most prominent writers about dyslexia and reading backwardness, and as Critchley, for instance, has attacked some of her opinions on occasion, her views are certainly worth noting, including her summary statement (1965) about the present position in the United Kingdom:

There is continuing controversy in Britain as to whether the condition termed "specific dyslexia" really exists; or whether all backwardness in reading can be attributed to environmental factors such as inadequate teaching and uncultured home backgrounds, or to emotional maladjustment. It seems probable that the 15-20 per cent of eleven-year-old children whom many surveys have found to be retarded by about two years in reading are in fact suffering from the effects of environmental handicaps. There is no doubt that children living in poor neighbourhoods, with parents quite uninterested in their school achievements, do show a lower average reading age than do those from better homes. Again, the teaching of reading, especially to children in junior schools, who have not learnt to read in the infants' schools, is often quite unsuitable. Many of the teachers of such children have little idea how to teach beginners. Yet it is equally true that not all children are affected by these environmental handicaps; nor have all backward readers, especially the severely retarded, suffered from them.

I have stressed throughout this book that the main confusion (in Britain and elsewhere) about the term dyslexia lies in the attempted definitions of the term rather than in disagreement as to its causes. For, unless it is agreed that dyslexia is a specific type of disability, with characteristic symptoms, it is a waste of time to attempt to discover causes.

To my way of thinking, no one—Critchley, Vernon, or anyone else—has made a tight case for the existence of dyslexia as a particular syndrome. Critchley says that only a small number of backward readers (even of severely backward readers) suffer from it, but cautions that diagnosis (not very clearly specified) is difficult; Hallgren says the same, admitting that some of the familial cases he was studying may have been borderline cases, but again leaving one in some doubt as to how the line is drawn with certainty. Now, Vernon (1965), while suggesting the existence of multi-causes and the existence of several kinds of dyslexia, confesses that not only is cause hard to establish in any particular case, as there is considerable overlap between the syndromes or groups of symptoms, but that nevertheless they possess certain specific features which do not seem to occur in non-dyslexic backward readers.

Vernon, as we have noted, is prepared to admit to a certain number of cases (of dyslexia) that do appear to possess a minor degree of brain damage "incurred during pregnancy, at birth, or shortly after".

She agrees, however, that an ordinary neurological examination will not always disclose these abnormalities, and that the E.E.G. pattern will only sometimes suggest them. At times this might be further supported by poor visual perception of complex forms (de Hirsch, 1954, quoted by Vernon, 1965), such as those of the Bender test, and by a poor showing in certain other tests such as the Object Assembly and Coding and Block Design sub-tests of the W.I.S.C., and in the Goodenough Draw-a-Man test; and, in my opinion, by unusualness of test solution pattern in some cases, as I mentioned earlier. There may be also, she says, some possible (but not certain) defect in speech and auditory perception, and some *possible* clumsiness, inattentiveness, impulsiveness, or sluggishness and perseveration.

In other words are we left with a mere theory as to the existence of specific dyslexia (or dyslexias)?

Not entirely. The crux of the position is indicated in the reference to a residue of cases with features "which do not seem to occur in non-dyslexic backward readers". In any reading clinic there will be cases of severe reading disability, showing signs of suspected minimal brain damage (or with a history which includes such damage) and others that do not; there will be cases of clumsiness and many that lack this; there will be cases of deficient or adverse environment, and many more from a "normal" environment. And there will sometimes be a small percentage of cases in any of the above categories or in other categories that bring the clinician up with a round start, that present a baffling picture and seem "different" from the other backward reading cases.

To say this is not to make any statement as to cause or specific symptoms—they vary quite a deal; it is merely to acknowledge the existence of these baffling cases whose main characteristic is *inability* to read or almost inability to read. One can understand why Dr Pringle Morgan, in the first case quoted in this book, was tempted to label his problem "congenital word-blindness". It is the same kind of bafflement which led a psychiatrist some months back, when referring one of his cases to me, to state, "I can't help feeling that he is one of these congenital dyslexics we read about".

Can Childhood Dyslexia Be Predicted?

This existence of baffling instances among the cases of severe reading retardation was in the mind of Dr John McLeod, until recently Director of the Remedial Education Centre, University of Queensland, when discussing the possibiliity of providing a means of predicting childhood dyslexia (1966), on the argument that the earlier we catch a dyslexic, the better is his chance of successful treatment; and that prevention, where such is possible, is even better still.

Obviously one can scarcely provide a test for potential dyslexics unless one admits that there is such a thing as dyslexia, or uses it to cover a clearly defined group of backward readers. McLeod, who is now with the University of Saskatchewan, is aware of the controversy over this term, but despite the "wilderness of contradictions" mentioned by Knud Hermann (1959) proceeds to identify dyslexia by pragmatic approach and then goes on to prepare a schedule for discovering the potential sufferers at an early age.

He notes the fact that many important writers in this field— among them Bender, Critchley, de Hersch, Hermann, Ingram, Money, Myklebust, Orton, Rabinovitch—have described cases of severe reading disability in which a characteristic pattern of symptoms can be sensed, but which is blurred by variability from patient to patient; he notes further that there are many literate parents from "normal" home environments whose children show a bewildering inability to learn to read, and yet these parents are not fools themselves and they know their children to be of good or above average common sense. He notes also the opinions of "recognised specialists" in the field (in other words clinicians in reading clinics) that there are reading problem children who seem to be different. On the basis of criteria of this kind, he is prepared to use the term dyslexia as having sufficient meaning for his purpose, so that the preparation of a test for culling out the younger children likely to become dyslexics is, he feels, justifiable.

He approaches the preparation of his *Dyslexia Schedule* in the same way that one might go about preparing a test of aptitude—for music, for mechanical ability, etc.—by obtaining the assistance of teachers and remedial workers, psychologists and others, in selecting a group of children believed by these workers to show signs of this difference—or, as he puts it, to be "dyslexia enriched" —then proposes that a schedule or test be devised containing items that (when taken as a whole, not necessarily item by item) fit the children in this group, and then to "sharpen" the instrument "by using it to predict further cases of dyslexia and observing its adequacy or inadequacy in doing so". In other words, using the group and then other groups, to *validate* the proposed items in the test.

In so far as the preparation of such a schedule does not make an assertion as to the exact nature or cause of dyslexia, and may in the long run predict potentially backward readers of varying kinds, the preparation of such a test seems to be desirable. It is not proposed here to deal in detail with the schedule but merely to remind readers of the work that has been done concerning it, and is still being done, in Queensland. The Dyslexia Schedule, together with a handbook for its use, and a School Entrance Check List, have now been published.

6

RELIEVING THE TENSIONS

Reference has been made to the difference of opinion between various schools of thought as to the importance of emotional difficulties to reading problems. It may be said, however, that a significant number of researchers and workers in this field hold the view that the emotional aspect of the problem is very important, perhaps of central importance, and attention must be paid to it if progress is to be made.

J. G. Lyle, in 1954, in an assessment of personality characteristics of fifty remedial reading cases, found as follows:

REJECTION FEELINGS

A critical score could be found above which most clinic children scored and below which most normal children scored. These feelings of rejection may be related to passive-dependent needs.

AGGRESSIVE REACTIONS

Clinic children gave more disguised aggressive reactions, and more uncontrolled emotional reactions than the normal child. The inference is not that these children are more aggressive, but that their aggression is unverbalised (unconscious).

REMEDIAL READING CHILDREN AND OTHER CLINICAL CHILDREN

There seems to be no difference between remedial reading children and other clinical children. The passive-dependent backward readers seem much the same as the passive-dependent enuretics, the passive-dependent stammerers, asthmatics, phobics, etc. It seems that reading retardation may be just another symptom of maladjustment and should not be regarded as a purely educational problem.

If this view is valid, and it is in accord with the opinions of many writers, as we have seen, it may suggest that best results will be achieved by treating the emotional problems first. Those who adhere most strongly to this point of view do place emphasis on treating the emotional problem *first,* claiming that a dramatic alleviation of the reading disability may result (and I have myself seen this take place in certain cases) once the patient has come to adopt tension-free patterns of behaviour.

Psychoanalytic writers, as we have noted, would be numbered among those who accept this claim, and we have referred to some of the things that Phyllis Blanchard has had to say about reading problems, emotional maladjustment and the psychodynamics of early childhood.

It is interesting to take a look at three cases reported by two psychoanalytically-oriented therapists (Sylvester and Kunst, 1943) as they illustrate three ways of approach to reading disabilities even when the prime importance of the emotional maladjustment is accepted for all three cases. In the first case, treatment was by both tutor and psychiatrist; in the second case, by tutor only; in the third case, by psychiatrist only.

Naturally, the interpretations given to various aspects of these cases and to the treatment and its apparent results, are of the kind one would expect from the analytic school; it is obvious also that the tutors were well versed in analytic lines of thinking and functioned partly as tutors and partly as therapists according to the exigencies that arose.

I do not think it is important here to question or seek to support psychoanalytic concepts, or to question whether or not interpretations given by the writers to various incidents or developments in the cases reported are valid; the main points seem to me to have been the recognition of emotional maladjustment in each case, the establishment of warm (if somewhat erratic) relations between therapist and patient and between tutor and patient, and the ultimate better adjustment (for whatever reason) of the patients both emotionally and in the sphere of reading.

In their search for reasons for disturbance of function—that is, the whys and wherefores of the emotional maladjustment and the reading disability—Sylvester and Kunst refer to "the behaviouristic manifestations of the instinctual tendencies . . . namely, the functions of incorporation, elimination and retention, and exploration". They assert that it is the emergence, interplay and fate of these functions that will ultimately determine an individual's capacity for adequate action and self-assertion.

Their theory would be that from early childhood, a child, with a view to maintaining his relations with his parents and so to guarantee his security, will make changes as needed, in the expression of his instinctual drives; sometimes these changes will assist in his development as an individual, but sometimes distortions and inhibitions of his drives will result in distortions to the personality that is developed.

They take it for granted that the reader will share their view that the experience of feeding and habit training will be reflected later in the child's character. They use the term "character" without moral implications—it refers merely to the type of person the individual ultimately becomes. The healthy development of the exploratory function with curiosity as to the nature and function of one's own body and that of others, and curiosity extended step by step beyond this to the wider world, will result, they would feel, in a capacity in the individual, at the right time, for abstract learning. On the other hand, interference with the healthy development of this function would manifest itself in ultimate emotional maladjustment, and especially in reading disability.

This is stating the analytic position a little more explicitly perhaps than Blanchard, for example, but it would be regarded as fairly representative analytic thought. It needs stating (or restating) if we are to understand the nuances of meaning in the cases that follow.

EXPLORATION AND READING

Sylvester and Kunst sum up this stated connection between development of the exploratory function and inclination or ability to read, as follows:

Given adequate intelligence the child must still have preserved the courage for active curiosity if he is to learn to read. The earliest objects of curiosity are the child's own body, and the immediate objects and persons of his early environment together with their mutual relationships. Curiosity as an aspect of the exploratory function is thus influenced by the earliest interpersonal experiences with all their emotional connotations. If these are traumatic the exploratory functions may become a danger to the child's security. This may occur in several ways. If the earlier functions of intake and elimination and retention have encountered unhealthy vicissitudes, or if the exploratory function itself has been traumatized, then curiosity, as an aggressive self-assertion becomes connected with anxiety toward those persons who exercise external control and, at the same time, are those on whom the child depends. On the other hand, if the exploratory function is over-indulged, the child is unable to manage the undue quantities of stimulation. In short, the learning process may become conditioned by anxiety which is generated by: (1) inadequate capacity for mastery; (2) fear of loss of love; (3) patient's own destructive threat toward the persons on whom he depends. The reading disability thus becomes a defence against anxiety which may be stimulated by curiosity.

These writers are of the opinion that total or near total inability to read is simply the outcome of severe anxiety resulting in a totally adverse reaction to books which are treated then by the child as "phobic objects" and persuasion will be no more effective in alleviating a "reading phobia" than it will be with other phobias, e.g. fear of closed spaces.

They state categorically that, with all their cases, whereas children have gone out of their way at the beginning of treatment to avoid books or cover them so that they cannot see them, with the alleviation of the basic problem or conflict, as anxiety diminishes, interest and ability in reading emerge.

They have drawn an interesting analogy between the way anxiety-ridden children may alter normal speed and rhythm of reading with the way some children behave when trying to deal with the fear of the dark. A reader may try to ease the anxiety by hesitating and pausing. He clings to the position he has reached and postpones making the next move to a new, unknown position, for as long as possible. Or he may attempt on occasion to rush the dangerous position by storm and shout. Thus may be seen the child who rushes headlong through a reading test or assignment. I have seen some tense children do this at testing sessions—rush through sixty questions in a test and get fifty-five wrong. Or on another occasion, sensing or knowing that there is light and escape just beyond the intervening darkness, he may take courage and tackle a reading book if told of the contents in advance.

Where a reading tutor was working with a child, regular discussions were held between tutor and psychiatrist, so that at all times the principles used would be within the framework of psychoanalytic concepts.

CASE I (Treatment by both tutor and psychiatrist)
Excessive Stimulation Inadequately Mastered, with Fear of Seduction as a Consequence

Boy, 6 years old; referral to clinic because of refusal to read at school, unruly behaviour generally, and in particular fire setting, and violence towards 3-year-old sister and towards mother.

Parents had displayed much uninhibited conduct in front of the children, with extreme display of love and hate; at the same time, because the boy displayed "apparent brilliance", he was pushed towards precocious maturity". · After a time the parents separated and the mother looked to the boy for support and comfort. She over-stimulated him in this way, but if he subsequently made approaches to her she would become violently angry.

There had been an earlier attempt at therapy by another psychiatrist at the clinic, but this had been discontinued when the boy was moved to the home of his grandparents, where he adjusted satisfactorily, except for a continued refusal to read. Eventually he had to return to his mother and his improved conduct now rapidly deteriorated again.

He was re-enrolled at the clinic and reading tutoring was attempted, although it was realised from the beginning that this in itself would be insufficient. At the first diagnostic session, he told the tutor that he could not read the test material because his mother's face was between him and what he was trying to read. He then paused and drew the tutor's face. His own poetry, which he recited, was full of expressions of loneliness and the need for protection, despite his swaggering behaviour on the surface. He became tense and anxious when finally induced to read (or attempt to read) some of the test words; some words he refused to try at all, and he also rejected the mirror reading test on the grounds that it was unknown to him and might make him "crazy".

It was soon apparent that continuance of formal tutoring was impossible, but he was developing an interpersonal relationship with the tutor which it was considered desirable to maintain, and on this basis he was seen by the tutor weekly for four months. He showed awareness of his mother's wish to rid herself of him and this brought an immediate reaction of extreme aggression towards the tutor, followed by regression to more dependent, infantile states in which he had to be dressed, cuddled and cared for. Phantasies appeared of an oral and anal nature, and this was interpreted on psychoanalytic lines as a retreat from his exploratory aggressive tendencies which had caused him such anxiety in the testing situation and had been avoided as indicated above.

At the end of this phase he sought the tutor's help in obtaining a kitten as a pet, then encouraged the tutor to display kindness and affection towards the kitten as proxy for himself, and while the tutor was so engaged, his exploratory tendencies reappeared, a little at a time, but now with less anxiety. He began by investigating the contents of a purse and a desk, and then even looked at some books that were in the room. Next he was able with little anxiety to ask openly questions about birth, at the same time demanding even more urgently the tutor's care for his kitten. He finally agreed to attend a summer camp, provided the tutor would "adopt" the kitten.

When the boy returned from the camp his mother placed him in a boarding school nearby and sessions of psychotherapy in a planned sense began. His symptoms changed, his aggressive behaviour dropped off as the tutor continued to give him unconditionally the interest and affection he craved. His curiosity was now manifest in a non-traumatic manner, and he accepted the "rules" of the boarding school that being "loved" depended on being "good"—that is, in behaving in a socially-acceptable way. He had learned through association with the tutor that love was valuable and it was worth his surrendering his previous pattern of behaviour to be sure of retaining it.

This meant repression of some urges which were now "acted out" in form of tics. As psychotherapy progressed he experienced periods of depression which alternated with what the clinic described as "seductive swaggering". He nicknamed himself "Bobby wise-eye, the boy who has seen too much and therefore does not want to live any more". He imagined (in phantasy) that his father was a great inventor who warned him not to look into one of the machines the father had invented, and which made fearful noises and moved about violently. But he does look into the machine and as a result has to run on through the years with closed eyes, wrecking the house as he runs, to stop the machine from catching him. He finally saves himself by pretending that he and not the father was the inventor of the machine, but that obviously it would be too dangerous for him to invent anything else.

This phantasy was interpreted as follows:

The phantasy is an obvious reference to the sado-masochistically conceived primal scene. It recapitulates his original reaction to the seductive home situation which had overwhelmed his capacity for healthy curiosity. His aggressive conduct, with hostility directed toward himself and the therapist, was met with the restrictions he seemed to invite. He seemed to wish for protection against the type of relationship he had had with his mother. The tics were a substitutive expression of his transference rage toward his mother who had on the one hand thwarted and on the other hand overstimulated him. A licking tic persisted until we had worked through his originally unsatisfied longing for the gratification of his dependent needs.

The outcome was satisfactory and the boy became happy at school and at play after six months' treatment and his reading, which had been three years retarded, was no longer a problem for him.

Whether or not the reader accepts the exact interpretation of his phantasy given above by the therapist, will depend on the extent to which he accepts an analytic viewpoint.

CASE II *(Treatment given by tutor only)*

Curiosity Inhibition, Through Fear of Rejection

Boy: 10 years old, one sister, 6 years younger. Referred to clinic because of infantile speech, childish behaviour and persistent eating problems.

Diagnostic tests showed that he had a severe reading problem, his average reading level being retarded by two years.

During parental interviews it became apparent that the father was indifferent to the boy and he was rejected by his mother. Both parents made a point of their strictness and unwillingness to "spoil" their son.

The mother had wanted a girl and had kept the little boy's hair in curls until he was nine months old, when she could no longer avoid cutting his hair. Her disappointment intensified as a result, and the boy became shy and withdrawn, thus conforming to the parental standards—seen but not heard.

With the birth of his sister, the boy showed extreme jealousy, and tried to master this by identifying with the baby; thus he began to talk in an infantile manner and there was an increase in his feeding difficulties. The outcome of this was even greater strictness and more punishment by his mother. He became desperate in his feeling of rejection and asked: "Why did you buy me if you think I am a bad boy?" He became stubborn—but in a meek sort of way—and was fearful if left alone. When he commenced school work he refused to read or to spell.

Habit-training (toilet, etc.) was slow and accomplished only by threats and punishment, and was an experience of fear for the boy. His sister's sex ensured for her a privileged position with the mother and this was traumatic for him. His curiosity—put in the form of timid questions about his mother's pregnancy—were silenced harshly by her, at once.

The therapists at the clinic interpreted the subsequent inhibition of the boy's curiosity as something he had to do, not only because the mother's attitude was so forbidding, but because he hoped magically to deny the existence of the coming child—the object of his questions. By denying its existence he could reduce the possibility of loss of love. As Sylvester and Kunst put it: "What he didn't know would not hurt him. His inhibition of curiosity as manifest in his reading defect, stems from this fact."

What he did read, in the tests, he read quickly (but not accurately) the impression being given that his main aim, when confronted with something to read, was to get through it, if he must, and be done with it. Remedial teaching lifted his accuracy level and his speed increased also, keeping ahead still, of his average reading level. Usually a child retarded in reading will show poor speed on a speed test, although, as we have mentioned, the child who rushes on, making many errors, is seen from time to time.

The boy showed strong curiosity about what other people were doing, but in a furtive way. He would come stealthily to the tutor's door and throw it open without warning, if the tutor was engaged with another patient. He would quickly flip through the desk calendar and even with the reading exercises would peep at them through a crack in his fingers, or cover the directions over and say that he would try to guess what he had to do. It seemed very painful to him to seek any form of knowledge openly.

In the fourth month he showed an increasing interest in science and asked many questions, the answers to which he obviously knew were contained in the next paragraphs. If the tutor allayed his fears by answering the questions before he was urged to read the paragraphs, his expected anxiety diminished, and the discrepancy between speed and accuracy disappeared completely.

He pressed on with his reading in science and expressed a desire for a microscope, which was provided for him. By now he had what was interpreted as "increasing courage to proceed with his investigations of things unknown". He even reported that in a dream he had invented a microscope lamp that was twice as powerful as the tutor's desk lamp.

The boy now expressed an interest in performing some experiments and he was permitted to do so. One of these in particular was seen by the clinic as "an acting out of the problem of his curiosity in relation to the gestation and birth of his sibling". It is described as follows:

The patient inserted a sprouted marigold seed into a slit made in the main stem of a begonia plant. He carefully bound the "wound" with a cloth which he thereafter kept wet for he feared the mother plant would not be able to keep the implanted seed sufficiently moist. He was afraid that his cutting operation on the begonia might cause it to die, but reassured himself with the thought that "plants can heal themselves". He calmly accepted the possibility suggested by the tutor that the inserted seed might not develop, but he hoped that the begonia would get new blossoms or would "at least change colour or something". He bore the inevitable failure very well. It was pointed out that even though in a sense the experiment had failed, he had learned something and there would be many more opportunities to learn.

He now seemed ready for open questions about conception and birth and asked the tutor directly. He then in a matter-of-fact manner compared the information given to him by the tutor with ideas of his own, and showed no anxiety. This was in marked contrast to the anxiety he had shown a year before when remedial reading had begun.

He maintained his speed of reading over the remaining months at the clinic, but brought his accuracy much closer to it. At the end of seventeen months his reading level was at about the expected average for sixth grade and his tutoring was terminated.

CASE III (Psychiatric Treatment Only)

Curiosity; Destructive Implications

Boy: 8 years old; enuresis, poor achievement at school; very restless.

He was in a subnormal room at school, but ability tests at the clinic showed that he was, in fact, of very superior intelligence. A complicating feature of his development was his mother's serious illness (severe heart disease) which frequently incapacitated her. Despite her illness, the mother had breast-fed him at her own insistence for ten months, and had suffered several major heart attacks during this time. He developed feeding difficulties after weaning, especially refusing to drink milk. As he passed through young childhood, periods of noisy hyperactivity alternated with apathetic inactivity or sluggishness. The psychiatrist gave as his opinion during treatment that there was a close connection between the hyperactivity and his mother's sick attacks.

He was given twenty-seven sessions of therapy and it is stated that his unevenness of mood disappeared, despite the mother's continuing heart attacks. At the time of reporting this case he had left the subnormal room at school and was progressing in normal grades. In ten months he had made a gain of 1.4 years in reading comprehension (in Gray's Oral Reading Test) and his courage to read had increased obviously.

His caution and apathy in his less active moods were explained to the clinician at beginning of treatment as "bad memory". And here, as one must expect in the psychoanalytic approach, an interpretation is interpolated:

To him bad memory meant: "I dare not know what I might do to my mother with my activity". Curiosity meant aggressively exploring the mother's body. In this boy, whose mother's body was already in such serious danger, this tendency had to be inhibited. The reading defect was an aspect of this blocking. It was the mother's ill health that he wanted to forget and deny by sending his memory "to play baseball". This aimed at relegating aggression into the innocuous world of phantasy. When his memory was lured back into the treatment room he played with a family of dolls. The mother doll refused to carry the baby since he might kick and push her from the table. To prevent such an accident, the patient tied the baby to the mother's arms.

When the boy became angry with the psychiatrist, and felt guilty because of this, his memory clouded over once again.

His reactions during treatment are interesting. The first time his mother became ill, he denied the fact. The second time he complained of "bad memory". Next he asked what would happen if the psychiatrist were pushed into the lake. This was followed by a request to be shown "deeds of speed and skill" in the drawing of such difficult objects as skeletons. He then assured himself of his own capabilities—"No amount of running and shouting could make him tired or ill". He proceeded to demonstrate this further by hammering and pounding away at a great rate and sought the participation of the psychiatrist in this also—this was something his mother could not do. He accidentally injured the psychiatrist with a hammer and at once became fearful and plunged into a bout of excited hyperactivity.

He was reassured regarding his fear and began a period of repairing and "fixing things like new". His tensions diminished and he suggested that he be transferred to a normal school class. He said he could now cope with such a grade, as his memory had improved.

The phantasies of this boy suggested that he was in the conflict situation of indulging in aggressive activity which he at the same time feared might endanger the survival of his mother. Curiosity too might endanger her survival. But the psychiatrist had assured him that she (the psychiatrist) could survive a fall into the lake, an injury with the hammer, and so on.

With his new freedom his curiosity emerged and he asked the

classical birth questions and showed interest spontaneously in a book dealing with this. This interest spread to other books.

These cases are given as examples by Sylvester and Kunst of their claim that the origin of a reading defect is "a single aspect of a more comprehensive disturbance in the evolution of psycho-biological functions". They conclude that "the disturbances in reading are disturbances of the exploratory function and that symptomatic treatment (that is, attacking the reading problem only) by pedagogical methods is not enough". They admit that remedial teaching *does* succeed, but maintain that "in such cases the tutor has met, intuitively, some of the psychological needs of the particular child".

Whether these cases demonstrate the validity of *psychoanalytic* principles is another matter, although the authors of the report would undoubtedly deny that the establishment of a warm relationship with the patient, and a recognition of his emotional needs is enough; a precise knowledge of these needs is necessary, they would say, and attention to them along psychoanalytic lines.

But here we must leave the matter.

7

CAN YOU HELP HIM TO READ?

The other evening I attended a function concerned with raising funds for a new wing to a local hospital, and passed the usual greetings with the young woman seated on my left. "I remember you," she said, "you gave the parents' committee a talk on dyslexia at the kindergarten a few years ago."

She was right, and I had found the parents and others that night just as interested in this question—almost paradox—of the near illiterate in a supposedly literate society, as I always do when speaking to groups on this topic. She went on to echo what I had heard so many others say so often. "I didn't think it possible that a problem like this could exist—children passing through school unable to read, or reading only with difficulty. But I had a niece who turned out to be a dyslexic when she reached third grade; she had to have help for about two years and finally was able to read."

Whether the niece she was talking about was a dyslexic or had any kind of severe reading problem is hard to say. I doubt it, or a further comment would have had to be added: "Even now, although much improved, she still has quite a deal of trouble with her reading."

It is interesting to note reasons given by parents at the interview that precedes testing in our clinic, for having sought an opinion and perhaps help for the child: "He didn't seem to read too badly, but he hasn't any interest in books"; or, "He stumbles about shockingly if you ask him to read anything to you"; or, "The teacher says something will have to be done about his reading now, it can't go any further"; or, "I feel that if he could read more quickly he could cope with his books better now that he is in secondary school"; or, "I had him along at the Guidance Bureau, and they said he is behind with his reading". And, of course, many variations of statements like these.

But, sooner or later, with statistical predictability, the parent replies: "Because he simply can't read; and if he writes anything down, it doesn't make sense."

I am not very interested in whether the boy or girl can read out with good intonation and correct pauses and all the rest, except in so far as this may (one way or another) be having an influence on the child's personal image of himself. Some attention is given in the normal course of clinic work to oral reading, but a speech-defect case would be referred to a speech therapist, and the parent with an eye to success at the next eisteddfod would be told that someone else must help her son or daughter.

My interest, and that of any reading consultant, would be to determine the extent to which one can *communicate* with the child through the written word, and what level of successful communication is desirable and possible for the client.

I have mentioned earlier a client of 14 years of age in our clinic, referred by a psychiatrist, and the sort of boy whose reading may aptly be described as "different" and his difficulty as severe. This boy will never read well; he will always make errors if called on to read *aloud*—at times even fairly simple sentences—and his spelling will always be "peculiar".

The mother's aim is to have him complete at least fourth year of secondary school, but the psychiatrist and I both know that this aim is unrealistic. The mother's feeling that the boy has laboured under a weight of inferiority feelings, and that if he leaves school at the statutory minimum age of 15 his feelings of inferiority will increase, may very well be true. Apparently he verbalises about himself quite a deal at home along the lines of, "I'm a dunderhead, it's no use worrying over me, I'm not going to get anywhere." But the chance that his inferiority feelings will increase, and perhaps more severely, if he stays on is equally likely, or, I think, more so. And this, despite the fact that the school at my request tries to avoid damaging competitive situations for him.

When considering a programme for this boy, one thing was clear. He would make no progress whatever until he altered, however slightly, his low self-esteem; it must be demonstrated to him, as incidentally as possible, that he *could* do some things with reading, there and then, that he had imagined himself unable to do. By ascertaining the sound combinations that he knew, for instance, and encouraging him to work out some words containing these combinations of sounds, for himself, or by using these sounds to build up words, himself, it was possible to let him see very quickly, that he could deal with some sight words the "shape" of which he did not recognise, in the first session. By encouraging him also to chat a little on some topic dear to his heart—his dog in this case—and then assisting him to write these things down and to add others without help, further progress could be made.

It goes without saying that the development of a warm personal relationship between the boy and the clinician was essential and this was accomplished successfully. Here was a boy who had begun to brood alone in his room, convinced that others couldn't be bothered with him (except his dog) and who came along to his first session with this sort of look on his face. That the way was going to be a little easier in the future became apparent a few sessions later, when he came to the door with a smile of greeting, began to take personal responsibility (unasked) for certain preparations during the session, such as pulling the blinds down, to darken the room before the tachistoscopic[9] exercises, plugging in the cord for the reading rate controller for his "eye exercises"[10] and setting the machine up for himself and so on.

It was important with this boy—and is important with most reading problem cases—that he should not feel that he had simply exchanged one classroom for another. Such children, must, of course, accept the fact that they are to carry out such assignments as are required of them—even school-exercise-type assignments at times when necessary—but the atmosphere should be unlike that of a classroom. "Sir" is discouraged as a form of address to me: either "Dr Hepworth", or often the non-address form of give and take conversation.

When decisions affecting a boy or girl have to be made, I like the client to have a definite part in arriving at the decisions. Although it is my belief in this particular case (but by no means in all cases) that to carry on for too long at school would be undesirable, I would not be prepared to force this opinion on the

---

9 A device for projecting controlled flashes of words, phrases and numbers on a screen at predetermined exposure times (e.g., from 1 second to 1/125 of a second.

10 Practice in underlining words, numbers, etc., matched to a key word or number to the left of the line and doing this quickly enough to avoid being overtaken by the "arm" of the machine moving down the page.

boy. I am quite prepared to be "directive"[11] in my therapy, in the sense of expressing an opinion as to what I feel is best, *if a boy or girl asks me to do so,* but I believe the boy's wishes or the girl's wishes and ideas should be carefully weighed and considered, if they are contrary to the clinician's ideas or those of school or family. An attempt should be made to ensure that the young client has both sides of the picture as he works his way to a decision. The pitfalls as well as the advantages should be clear to him.

By the way, where more than one person—professional or family or both—is "dealing with" a client, for instance a reading consultant and a psychiatrist, the impression should not be given (and in fact it should not be so) that there is any "ganging-up" on the client; some free-flow of ideas and information may be necessary, but confidence should never be betrayed if ultimate good is to be achieved in a severe reading problem case or in any other problem case. A boy could hardly arrive at a personal decision if he felt that sheer weight of numbers was against him.

This client is a boy of average ability as measured on a nonverbal intelligence test, but he has a curious inability to pronounce clearly certain words (even some in his everyday vocabulary, including the name of his own country, which he pronounces "Australa"), or repeat certain words correctly after the clinician has said them. I can't see any deep significance in the words mispronounced, as a Freudian might—they don't seem to be related in form or idea to one another as a group, or to any special stage or function in the psycho-sexual development of the individual. Some of the syllables mispronounced or omitted in some words may be included and correctly pronounced when they appear in other words, or at other times. He gives a strong impression to the clinician that he cannot *hear* the sounds in some words when they are spoken to him, but can hear them in other words.

If he starts to read for "cream" the sound "cl" he may change to a "cr" sound if this is pointed out to him, but he will soon be back to the "cl" once again. Anything more difficult than to demonstrate long and short vowels to him (in the simplest terms) I cannot imagine and when he has it for, say, "od-ode", he will not have it for "at-ate" or "ut-ute" and so on.

---

11 As opposed to so-called non-directive therapy or counselling where an almost artificial attempt is made by the therapist to avoid giving directions or advice of any kind. Rogers is the name best known in this field.

When he came along first, he didn't just "mix up" the "b's" with the "d's"—he almost *always* said "b" for "d" and "d" for "b".

This boy is Jewish and for a time attended a Jewish school. Whether the right-to-left approach of the simple Hebrew he had there had any effect on his reading disability, it is hard to say, but I doubt it; his inability to repeat heard sounds at times, and his lack of connection between sound and visual symbol, go back, I understand, to the beginning of his reading at school, before "other language" problems had time to affect him.

He can now extract quite a deal of information for himself, even from reasonably difficult books (such as one dealing with the Californian gold rushes of the last century) *especially if he chooses the book for himself.* If he insists on saying "avisable" for "advisable" if asked to read the word or always reads "can not" for "can't", it is still success for him, as it does not interfere with the *communication* through reading, which at first, for him, was almost nil.

He may know quite well that "Mrs Carter" is the mother of "John Carter" in a story, but may read, "Miss". This is no problem for him, but it would interfere with communication to others and so is more needful of correction.

I have attempted to illustrate by reference to this boy's case the way in which a goal that is realistic and helpful has to be set for each client. This goal may correspond with the vague (or firm) notions that a parent has in mind, or it may not. It is highly desirable that we should all spell perfectly—but none of us does and many who would be conceded by everyone to be quite literate or even highly educated, have more than a little difficulty with their spelling. Yet this may be a yardstick by which a boy or girl's reading proficiency will be measured by a parent or teacher. Some children can be encouraged by improved visual means, or improved listening skills, or compilation of alphabetically arranged personal error cards[12] and in other ways, to greatly improve their spelling, but in this boy's case spelling improvement will be both slight and slow. So, for his programme, spelling improvement is not high on the list. Nor is exact oral reading. The success or failure of his reading assistance would be judged

---

[12] My spelling errors and errors in meaning are different from yours, and yours from those of the person next door. It is no use, therefore, *teaching* long lists of identical spellings and meanings to everyone, for our needs differ so widely.

more along these lines: once he could not communicate through reading or be communicated with by reading; if now (as is the case) he can do this to some extent, the programme is for him satisfactory and the progress positive. If in himself there is evidence of a new spark of life and self-esteem (as there is), the progress is even more satisfactory.

Our task is to continue to narrow the gap between ability and performance as far as possible, but accept the fact that there very likely always will be *a* gap, and help the boy to find a new means of measuring himself and of accepting himself as he is likely to be.

A boy with a problem such as the one I have just described must of necessity receive individual assistance, but others with problems less dramatic and severe benefit quite well from participation in a small group, providing the individuals in the group (4 to 8) are working on individual programmes, differing in each case a little from every other one. If the need for absolute and continuous individual assistance is not so great as to mitigate against progress within a group, the presence of others may reassure a boy that he is not unique in his problem and that as the others hope to progress, so might he hope also.

The heading of this chapter, "Can you help him to read?", was chosen because it is a question asked rather anxiously by parents (and teachers) quite often. In reply I usually point out that we are dealing with human beings, and so an unqualified "yes" could be given only by a charlatan. I then add, however, that as a gain in reading level and in personality is the normal outcome of a remedial reading programme under a properly trained and qualified clinician, even with severe cases such as the one outlined above, there is no reason to believe that in the case about whom the parent is asking the question, the outcome will be other than successful.

This necessitates an adequate diagnostic session and an interpretation of results and realistic goals to the parents before therapy or treatment or the remedial programme—call it what you will—begins.

All-Round Improvement

When a boy or girl is brought for consultation and assistance to a reading clinic, the most obvious criterion of success after a time will be the extent to which the client has raised his reading levels. But it is gratifying for a clinician to be told that an "all-round" improvement has been apparent to parents and teachers, and this kind of comment is not infrequent. Of many examples that could be given I have in mind a lawyer's son; he is fourteen years old, I.Q. in the "better half of normal"—that is, between 100 and 110—who was behind not only in reading, but in much of his school work besides, and who was also labouring under a psychological disadvantage; in other words, he was emotionally maladjusted. The boy was tall and gangling, with glasses, and a somewhat pedantic way of speaking, "Please, shall I obtain a marker for my eye exercises now?" Naturally this made him a fairly easy mark for the "teasers" at school, who made him the butt of their humour.

It might be expected that the lad would be adversely affected emotionally by this situation, and this was so. It was not in the sense of withdrawal, however, but in a strong drive to make friends, with aggression taking over when the inevitable failures occurred. His inability to make friends easily did not daunt him as might be the case with some others; it simply narrowed the field, as it were, so that he finished up with a small group of friends, poor readers and poor adjusters, as he was.

It was by being the "same" as this small group that ensured him of their friendship, and mitigated also against any special wish he might otherwise have had to improve his reading level and join the ranks of the "readers" instead of remaining one of the "non-readers". For it was clear even at the initial interview and diagnostic appraisal session that he felt more sure of success in friendship-making in the non-reading same-as-he group, than in the school at large. Had he not proven that he *could* make friends among the non-readers, and was there not a possibility that he might *not* succeed in catching up with the readers or becoming like them? And to become like them he would have to improve not only in his reading performance, but somehow to have teachers and boys regard him differently—less of a joke and a clown. Give a dog a "bad" name and it would take more than a few upward movements of reading level to rid him of it.

And yet, he did improve. Slowly at first—almost imperceptibly. But in the third term of assistance (one two-hour session per week), his speed of reading increased by nearly five times—from about 170 words per minute, to about 850 words per minute—and his comprehension was mainly 90-100 per cent on the after-reading checks, despite the fact that he was now reading material of a much higher level of difficulty.

Just about the time that this upsurge began, I received a 'phone call from his mother, telling me that her son would be returning for the third term as I had advised. "He is a new boy," she said, "showing all-round improvement. His examination results are better, his 'understanding' is better and he has a much improved personal outlook." She added that the boy himself attributed much of this to participation in the reading programme and was keen to return for term three.

I might add that he was also keen for his best friend (non-reader) who had been tested by me, to join also. His friend did join and the earlier client has taken the self-imposed responsibility of keeping an eye on him—explaining the whys and wherefores of certain exercises, etc.—in the early stages.

Despite the fact that this client had quite a deal to gain, in a way, from remaining a poor-reader in a poor-reading group, and so being sure of acceptance by someone, there were facets of his personality and background that pointed in other directions; he was assiduous in his attention to out-of-clinic assignments ("home-work" between sessions); he was, usually, "friendly" to the clinician and would chat as an equal at times. He had no sibling rivalry problem, and although his mother was perhaps a little over-anxious for him, she was on the whole able to take a reasonably objective view of his disability and his chances of a successful outcome. Finally, he could go on to new groups and not leave all his friends behind him—he took at least one of them along, as it were, with him.

As the lad increased his reading speed and comprehension, his inter-session reading assignments increased in volume and variety, with good effect on his general knowledge, which had been poor.

Other Ways Of Dealing With The Problem

The author agrees with Critchley's expressed view on treatment (stated here in somewhat over-simplified form), namely, that providing the programme is intense and interesting, the exact nature of it is not critical. The programme must be *personal*— that is, both tailored to the young client's needs and such that he or she can perceive that the tutor is genuinely interested in him or her as a person. I believe that the personality of the tutor is important also. Some people easily and immediately "click" with children and the grounds for a warm relationship are readily established.

The bibliography at the end of this book contains many refer-

ences which include sections (in some cases the whole volume)
dealing with method. They all have something to offer, even where
the method suggested arises directly from a one-school type of
thinking. It would be an almost overwhelming task to set down
the detailed remedial methods that have been put forward by
various writers, and the reader will want, in any case, to consult
several of them himself, if he is a student or a teacher particularly.

Two books that will, I feel, be found especially helpful are:
The Disabled Reader . . . Education of the Dyslexic Child
(edited by John Money), John Hopkins Press, Baltimore, 1966; and
The Second International Reading Symposium, by J. Downing
and Amy L. Brown, Cassell, London, 1967.

These books are not of course limited to method, but with reading and reading problems generally. But quite a deal is said about
method and, importantly as I see it, from many points of view.
For example, the Money book contains thirteen chapters written
expecially for it by invited contributors and four chapters by
authors whose work was published earlier.

Coming closer to home, the *Proceedings, Dyslexia Symposium,
Melbourne,* edited by Freda Hooper and R. N. Harrison and
published by The Australian College of Speech Therapists, Melbourne (1968), gives striking evidence of the heterogeniety of
interest in this problem, for so many and varied professions were
represented by the speakers—speech therapists, educationalists,
psychologists, neurologists, opthalmologists, psychiatrists and
others. Here again, the aim and purpose of the Symposium was
not directed exclusively, or even mainly, to method, but method
was included in many of the papers read there and reported in the
Proceedings. Mrs Freda Hooper (Speech Therapist), in her paper,
Statement of the Problem, sees a relationship between dyslexia
and "cluttering", a disorder characterised by rapid a-rhythmic
speech; Dr Marianne Frostig, *Theory and Research Findings Concerning Learning Disturbances,* emphasised the need to take individual differences into account; while Dr Marie Neale, *Patterns
of Dyslexia: Predictive Studies and Early Intervention,* stressed
the importance of non-directive behaviour modification.

As further examples of variety of approach, the reader may care
to consult also: Dr Alfred Tomatis, whose insistence on the importance of listening (to the acquisition of language and of reading)
goes far beyond a mere emphasis on auditory skills; Joan K. Atkinson, Kathleen J. Cochrane and J. Elkins of the Fred and Eleanor
Schonell Educational Research Centre, University of Queensland—

especially the case of "Brian T."; the Dr Grace M. Fernald and Helen B. Keller method (and J. Louis Cooper's suggested adaptation of this method). For all these and others, see the bibliography appended.

As a matter of interest and further illustration of variety of theory and approach to therapy, but *not* as an alternative to consultation of the references themselves, I shall now give a brief resumé of three of the papers read at the Symposium, and because of its almost startling novelty and perhaps somewhat less ease of consultation, the theory and method put forward by Dr Tomatis.

The Clutterer and the Dyslexic

Mrs Freda Hooper, Consultant Speech Therapist at the Coonac Rehabilitation Centre and Honorary Speech Consultant at the Royal Melbourne Hospital, draws attention to a speech disorder which she refers to as "cluttering"—and which she describes as a "disorder characterised by rapid, a-rhythmic speech", and with the words tumbling over one another. "Even voice quality can suffer. Pauses for breath are usually disregarded with the result the text is often incomprehensible to both reader and listener. Rate of acceleration within longer words increases in proportion to the number of syllables. The clutterer, who is usually unaware of his disorder, improves in performance when his attention is drawn to it." Her mental picture of a clutterer is of a patient "bursting into the Speech Therapy Clinic, usually bumping into someone, or something, before reaching the chair. Often restless, impulsive and gauche it is easy to understand why he irritates his fellows and teachers." She quotes studies[13] which seem to support Orton's view (1937) that a "clutterer is a double first-cousin to a dyslexic patient". Dysgraphia, or deficiency in writing, is also a concomitant of cluttering.

Mrs Hooper says that she brought up the question of cluttering and discussed the disorder in some detail because her own experience with clutterers had convinced her that the perceptual and auditory disturbances so often seen in such patients are responsible for their difficulties in reading and writing.

She posed the question, then, whether dyslexia was, perhaps, part of the cluttering syndrome. For the disorder seems to affect

---

[13] For example, that conducted by George Shepherd and Dr Arnold at the National Hospital for Speech Disorders, New York, 1960.

so many of the channels of communication—"speaking, reading, writing, rhythm, musical ability and behaviour in general".[14]

Mrs Hooper mentions the case of a boy, Bill, referred to an Education Department therapist. Testing revealed that the dyslexia difficulty was minimal and therapy concentrated on establishing confidence in the boy to deal with his cluttering problem, while at the same time offering advice concerning seeking extra assistance for his weaker school subjects. "Improvement has been marked within a matter of weeks, and end of the year results at school are better than usual."

So in at least some cases of dyslexia, where cluttering is also present, treatment is directed mainly towards the alleviation of the cluttering with faith that there will be alleviation of the dyslexic problems as a result, and this does seem to take place, at times.

Naturally one's mind turns from cure to prevention, or at least to early diagnosis, and the question is raised whether such early diagnosis with a boy like Bill, *before* he has encountered failure and is still able to benefit from a programme designed to meet his neurophysiological needs, would minimise or even prevent the disorder? This would necessitate the introduction of special training for teachers or intending teachers of young children to give them a deeper knowledge of the processes involved in the development of reading and writing skills.

If I am quoting Mrs Hooper correctly, I believe she sees value in a joint threefold approach of speech therapist, teacher and psychologist, both in cases of what she believes are developmental dyslexia (presumably of the Critchley type) and cases of "acquired dyslexia", including, or perhaps consisting entirely of, brain-injured patients who have suffered a breakdown in reading skill, or impaired facility to develop reading skills.

With A. E. Tansley,[15] she would seem to feel that "reading difficulty is a symptom rather than a clinical entity". But, she asks, "A symptom of what?"

Depending on the way we answer this question will we prescribe a programme of therapy or treatment in any particular case.

Many And Varied Approaches

Dr Marianne Frostig, Ph.D., Director of the Marianne Frostig Center of Educational Therapy, Los Angeles, who was one of the

---

14 The author has mentioned earlier personal observations of "jerkiness" of speech in some cases of serious reading disability.

15 *Reading and Remedial Reading.* Routledge, Kegan Paul. 1967.

principal speakers at the Melbourne Symposium, summed up the
fact of individual differences (at least as far as the dyslexics themselves are concerned). She said:

No one kind of teaching materials, methods or curricula is the best
approach for all the children in a classroom. The ways in which
children learn vary greatly, and teaching techniques must take individual differences into account . . . In each classroom there will be
children with reading difficulties. A single method cannot be best for
all these children.

Dr Frostig goes on, however, to draw attention to a number
of broad areas where difficulty is most likely to be encountered
and with which the clinician or tutor must deal. She believes
that dyslexic children frequently are found to have difficulties
in the social and emotional spheres and developmental lags in
sensory-motor, perceptual, linguistic and/or higher thought processes. Specific ability training should be provided in cases of
specific disabilities in each developmental area.

Lack of academic progress—that is, the extent to which a
child is "behind" the expected level of achievement—is, naturally, of considerable concern to the teacher. In helping the child
to overcome this lag, the developmental difficulties that he shows
must be taken into account. If the initial evaluation or diagnosis
has been correctly done, it should be possible to sum up both his
strengths and his weaknesses and so to determine the best way
to help him. As an example she cites the child who displays severe
visual perception disabilities. "He can be taught new content
orally or by means of a tape recorder, while at the same time
receiving carefully programmed training in visual perception."
Gradually the supplementary methods would be withdrawn from
the programme until he is finally able to master the material
necessary for him by reading books which are suited to his age
level.

With needs relating directly to *emotional and social development* psychotherapy or counselling may be required—for the
child and, perhaps, parents also. However, this will not always
be necessary. The teacher in his handling of classroom and play-
ground activities and in guiding the interactions of the children
has an opportunity to establish a satisfactory relationship with
them and to provide therapy in doing so. The teacher must guide
the child, "help him to succeed, set limits, accept his feelings
whether positive or negative". He must be assured of the teacher's
continual attention, concern and interest. Not only must the
teacher help the children under his care, but they must be

encouraged to help and support each other. They should all share in the daily tasks, and feel that, no matter what their contributions may be, they are respected.

In short, the classroom should provide a *therapeutic atmosphere*.

Some children who are *disorganized, impulsive, and hyperactive* are unable to focus attention at will or to follow a "sequence of stimuli". These disturbances, she says, are more global and pervasive and cannot be pruned down specifically to some developmental lag. She suggests three main approaches to reduce such global symptoms: "Focusing attention, providing structure, and promoting ego growth by reducing anxiety."

1. *Focusing Attention*. This can be achieved in two ways—by stimulus reduction (e.g., use of bare walls, masked windows, cubicles, a curtailed programme, etc.) or by stimulus accentuation —use of colour, boundaries, movement so that a stimulus will stand out from other stimuli. Dr Frostig adds that she uses stimulus reduction "sparingly".

2. *Providing Structure*. For instance, in behaviour, by consistency in use of basic rules of conduct in the classroom; or through tasks involving sequences of action (e.g., buttoning a coat or solving a problem in arithmetic, where careful analysis is carried out, and progression is through a succession of small, taught steps; and exercises in structuring time, by reference to events in the past—both recent and more distant—and by reference to future actions, attention to lapsed time, and so on.

3. *Ego Growth Through Reduction of Anxiety*. By a good relationship between teacher and child and by promotion of reassuring contacts among the pupils, as suggested above, and by gearing tasks to the child's abilities. I have mentioned earlier in the book the importance of avoiding unnecessary failure experiences. An immediate positive reaction to the child's endeavours is important. Appropriate rewards—that is, rewards suitable to this level of development (maturity) and to his needs, as far as these are known. Praise and stars may be as effective as more material rewards.[16]

Dr Frostig reminds us of the importance of collecting the child's work and recording his progress, as a graphic illustration to him of what he has accomplished.

---

[16] Learning theorists have shown that human subjects will often respond quite well in tasks if the only reward they receive is a one-word acknowledgement that they have given the correct answer.

It is not possible, nor is it my intention, to cover in detail all or any of the Symposium papers—they can be read, in the Proceedings, by those interested. However, I should like to mention Professor Marie Neale, presently Professor of Special Education at Monash University, formerly a Senior Lecturer in Education, University of Sydney and (Hon.) Psychologist at the Neurology Outpatients' Clinic, Royal Alexandria Hospital for Children, Camperdown, N.S.W. Her paper, *Patterns of Dyslexia . . . Predictive Studies and Early Intervention,* was concerned, as the title suggests, with several aspects of the problem, but one of them in particular, early intervention, necessitated a discussion of method.

To attempt prediction of possible dyslexia, it is obvious that Professor Neale cannot define dyslexia solely in terms of the extent to which a child may be behind the reading level of similar age and grade. Such an approach would mean waiting until the child had begun his school life. She *is,* of course, interested in those children who fail to acquire adequate skills in reading, spelling and written expression, and in ways of assisting them. Here we shall note what she has to say about firstly discovering the pre-school child who is a potential dyslexic,[17] and, having discovered him, taking measures to prevent the later occurrence of the problem. Although this is not a statement of treatment method for the dyslexic at school, it is appropriate to mention it here, as it is a treatment method for the factors that she considers lie behind many of the reading problems encountered at school.

Professor Neale looks for "imbalance in individual development"—that is, areas of development in the child that appear to be lagging behind the development of other areas in the same child. Even so, no attempt is made to stimulate directly the areas that are believed to be lagging, but to "involve the child in a variety of ways", and she labels the method of doing this as "non-directive behaviour modification". Following, she says, are some of the ways by which she approaches this:

(a) Play with a supervisor who enlarges, dramatizes and describes the activity to draw the child totally into the game.

(b) Games and activities that are carefully graded for progression in skilled co-ordination.

(c) Perceptual training, e.g., copying a particular style of action

---

[17] See McLeod's approach to prediction of childhood dyslexia in Chapter 5.

in detail, finding the missing pieces in a building construction (3 dimensions), making or copying of plans, maps, etc., noticing changes in the room, positions of objects, animals, and pictures, dramatization and puppetry.

(*d*) Listening to his/her own voice and other noises on the Language Master, piano and tape recorder. Looking at self in the mirror with eye-tracking exercises.

(*e*) Creating surprises, i.e., finding new ways to play with old equipment; suggesting novel uses for utensils and objects; dreaming up new characters for familiar animals.

(*f*) Extending the range of general experiences.

She stressed that no prescriptive lesson be given to apply generally, partly because children differ so fundamentally, one from another, "in organizing visual stimuli".

The Importance Of Hearing

As promised, I shall now give a summary of what I believe to be the main points in Dr Tomatis's hearing method of approach to therapy.

A great deal of attention has been paid to the importance of auditory discrimination and to the acquisition of auditory, visual and motor skills in the development of reading facility. Various tests, exercises and even machines have been devised to promote the acquisition of these skills by the learning child. It is not surprising, therefore, to read a statement by a French authority, Dr Alfred Tomatis (1969), in a monograph entitled "Dyslexia", that auditory skills are important to the young reader, but it is arresting to have him assert categorically that dyslexia is a disorder of auditory origin.

To be able to write, he says, is nothing else but to register the signs, which on the whole, is just what a magnetic tape does . . . A written sign in itself is nothing else but a coded sign to be reproduced.

Tomatis emphasises as a basic for the treatment he later prescribes, the importance to the developing foetus of the *sound* of the *mother's* voice as it is heard *in utero*.

The child at birth is then almost immediately surrounded by the world of air to which he has to adapt, so very different from the liquid bath he has just left; the newborn hears the same voice he had experienced for so long in the depths of uterine darkness. It is certainly different, but he recognises the inflexions, the rhythm, and from now on he will open his ear to listen to this new way of communication, tracing it back to the Nirvana which he has just lost.

As the child grows older he will still retain messages, secretly coded, "oriented to his mother". But he is now in a new world and so is "obliged to absorb conventional and social language which represents his father's attitudes".

Tomatis then goes on to discuss the development of the growing child and the interaction of his wishes with his relationship to his parents. Any difficulty met along the way, interfering with this interaction, "will prevent maturation for one or more of the processes which the ear must acquire to take its place of significance in the structuring of the language".

Tomatis would hold that dyslexia is an outcome of this interference, but that the problem is not limited to reading.

It embraces all types of relationship, indeed everything that has to be integrated. The one who is affected by "dyslexia" not only does not know how to read, but he cannot apprehend the world he lives in, normally, nor can he explain it correctly. He does not use the same coding.

In keeping with his theory as to the importance of listening, his diagnostic procedures involve careful but rather subjective attention to the postures of the child while he is listening to the examiner and to the postures also that he adopts while speaking to the examiner, for the words used, and the manner of using them reflect the underlying feeling that accompanies them.

Following the clinical observation tests, various physical and psychometric tests are administered. Vision is important and hearing, of course, is tested with thoroughness. If deafness is revealed, Tomatis gives weight to possible psychological factors and to listening deficiencies during the developmental period.

Treatment By Auditory Methods

In essence, it could be said that the treatment prescribed by Dr Tomatis consists in helping the young patient to acquire ways of using his ear "as an apparatus capable of listening".

We could scarcely quarrel with this aim, stated in general terms. Tomatis goes on to prescribe a therapeutic programme which seeks to recreate the wish to communicate, and is based directly on his theory of auditory development in the womb and later.

Treatment, he says, for benign cases is necessary for about three months: twelve months for severe cases. Sessions of approximately one half-hour each may take place perhaps every second day; or on one day per week for up to three weeks, with two or three sessions in the day.

1. *The period of "filtered sounds".* Auditory conditioning begins with sound or with the voice, which is passed through the electronic filters to make it identical with the sound the patient would hear if he were listening *through layers of water,* and hearing the maternal voice. Looking back to the pre-birth days, in other words.

2. *The 'performing'.* This stage calls for the intervention of a "THIRD PERSON", usually a physician or a psychologist. That is, someone additional to the child himself and to the mother.

3. *The 'training'.* Thus is the final stage. By the time it is reached, the patient is left to himself.

Later he can take educational help from what is referred to as the "OTHER", or outside person.

In other words, Tomatis places the greatest emphasis on the specialist training prior to the commencement of the educational programme, not on the educational programme itself. The success of the latter will depend on the thoroughness and faithfulness with which the hearing programme has been carried out.

To do justice, in summary form, to reporting a revolutionary concept of dyslexia such as that proposed by Dr Tomatis, is difficult, if not impossible. Questions naturally arise in one's mind—the apparent subjectivity of assessment in diagnosis, and the problem that might confront the clinician if the mother were dead or not otherwise available in the treatment period. For it is the mother's voice that the child hears filtered through the water, to simulate more specifically the "in utero" situation.

Obviously, for the interested student, perusal of the monograph itself is essential as a first step towards evaluating the concept.

8

RESULTS OF PERSONAL RES EARCH

The Emotions and Family Influence in 200 Reading Disability Cases

It was indicated early in the book that this discussion of reading disability stems from research carried out by the author by analysis of the case records of children and adolescents who have consulted him and have received reading clinic assistance during the past decade. It is not appropriate here to reproduce the statistical tables and calculations from that study, but a summary of the findings will be given. Also six cases will be included as examples of the two hundred that were the subject of the study.

The cases were divided into two groups. One hundred were "familials" . . . that is, cases with a brother or sister (sometimes two or more) in the clinic at the same time, or at other times; the second hundred were "non-familials" . . . that is, they had no known relative or relatives of any kind who had received treatment here or elsewhere, for reading disability, nor were any reported to have a sibling (or other relations) said to be dyslexic, or otherwise poor at reading.

The familial cases were chosen for study by random selection through the files, and without reference to sex, age, I.Q., or length of treatment in the clinic. An attempt was made to spread the selection throughout the alphabet, as far as possible. In most instances it happens that treatment ranged from one to three school terms of one two-hour session per week (or the equivalent in holiday sessions), and in most cases the I.Q. was 90 and upwards, as this is not a clinic for mentally retarded children.

Method of selection of the non-familials was to take at random about the same number of cases beginning with a particular letter as was selected for the familials.

The hypothesis which it was proposed to test in the course of the study, and which was formulated from observation in clinical practice, was as follows:

That there is a relationship between familial influences, emotional maladjustment and reading disabilities. In suggesting that there was a relationship between these factors, no assertion was made as to their nature . . . that is, for example, as to whether family influence is to be construed as hereditary influence or environmental influence or both. I have already pointed out in the chapter on heredity (Hallgren's study) that children in the one family share a similar environment, in many respects.

METHOD

The two hundred cases were assessed in terms of:

(*a*) Presence or absence of a family history of reading disability.

(*b*) Severity or otherwise of such emotional maladjustment as was present in particular cases.

(*c*) The severity or otherwise of the reading disability.

(*d*) The extent to which (if at all) the reading problem was ameliorated as a result of treatment.

Severity or mildness of reading disability was assessed by the use of standardised tests[18] during diagnostic appraisal sessions. The *criterion of reading disability* was the failure of a client to obtain a score *at least* equal to that expected of the "average" pupil of his age or grade, as I have described with reference to school surveys.[19] The *criterion of severity or mildness of reading disability* was the discrepancy exhibited between ability level of the client as revealed by the administration of a suitable I.Q. test or tests, and performance level as revealed on the reading tests.

The presence, absence and degree of severity of emotional problems was assessed in terms of various criteria, including clinical observation during the initial testing sessions and during the remedial period. Consideration was also given to information gained during interviews with the parents and to comments made by the parents during the remedial period or after its

---

18 Both 'reading level' tests and diagnostic tests.
19 Chapter 1.

termination. Sometimes also a child would come armed with a referral note from a psychologist or psychiatrist, or from a medical practitioner, school counsellor or teacher, with special reference, perhaps, to the possible presence of emotional or behavioural problems. The way a child did his tests during the diagnostic session—that is, the pattern of correct and incorrect answers he displayed—was also revealing, in many instances.

Improvement was assessed in terms of scores in follow-up testing sessions, by an evaluation of session record cards and by comments of parents and/or teachers, psychologists, psychiatrists and so on, where such were forthcoming.

Finally, reading improvement and emotional improvement were compared between the two groups . . . the familials and the non-familials.

In determining the programme of remedial treatment, heed was paid to the clinical observation and judgments made in the diagnostic appraisal sessions as well as to the test results. Again, when deciding whether the time had arrived for cessation of treatment, further observations and judgments were made and tests administered where appropriate. Attention was given also to comments by the client as well as by close associates of him.

Statements by the clients themselves are always enlightening. For example, a lad of seventeen, when talking to me recently said, "I never passed an examination in my life until I came to the clinic," and went on to discuss maturely his plans for entry to a tertiary institution, and clearly was capable of doing so. My mind went back to the extremely tense boy who had frequent nightmares, who he once was.

As an example of a parent's comments, one could cite the remarks of a mother that, apart from the general settling down of her son now at school, compared with a very poor record earlier, she could hardly recognise him for the same person about the house.

Comments made at the diagnostic interview by another mother about her son, referred by a psychiatrist as "probably a congenital dyslexic", were to the effect that he completely bewildered her. The remarks written on his school report (after three terms) by his headmaster were: "There is good reason to congratulate him on how much he has achieved—well done". The psychiatrist's note was: "Significant progress". The mother's new statement was: "He has amazed me at times recently with the things he has read out".

These instances are included (and many more could have been added, both from diagnostic interviews and from after-treatment statements) to show some of the things that must be taken into consideration in the assessment of the problem and of the outcome of treatment.

FINDINGS FROM THE STUDY[20]

The hypothesis was confirmed by the study which showed that there is a relationship between reading disability, emotional mal-adjustment and familial influence, and that this relationship affects the prognosis, or prospect of successful treatment in a given case.

In other words, both the reading problem and the emotional difficulty occur side by side in the one individual more often when he comes from a family with a history of reading problems. Also, in both the familial and in the non-familial cases, reading improvement and emotional improvement occur together much more frequently than one would expect from chance.

The study leaves unsettled the question as to whether the familial influence is genetic (hereditary) or environmental.

What seems at first sight to be a surprising conclusion is the fact that no connection was indicated between reading improvement and length of stay in the clinic, for both the familial instances and the non-familial instances. This is less surprising, however, when it is noted that almost always parents associated with the clinic continue the enrolment of their children until results of re-tests or other forms of re-assessment indicate that sufficient improvement for cessation of treatment has taken place.

In other words, this finding is not the same thing as saying that a client could be removed from treatment at any time, perhaps capriciously, with no fear of detriment to improvement. Indeed, the length of stay needs of one client may differ substantially from those of another.

It was shown that the most important environmental factor in both emotional improvement and reading improvement was therapy . . . that is, remedial assistance with the needs of the total child kept in mind.

The ability level of the child (I.Q.) bore little relationship to outcome with the familial group. This does not mean that the

---

[20] For the student I shall add (without explanation) that the statistical techniques employed were tetrachoric correlation and biserial correlation, depending on the particular material being considered at various points of the study.

lower ability clients in this group had opportunity for the *same extent* of reading improvement as those with higher ability. It simply means that their lower ability did not preclude them from achieving a satisfactory reading improvement, although this *may* be less substantial than might eventuate with a higher I.Q. case; however, this latter surmise is not specifically indicated in the results. Among the non-familial cases, I.Q. and degree of reading improvement did appear to be positively related, the brighter ones achieving a greater degree of success than the others. It is not clear why the two groups differed in this regard, but the study was not designed to explore this in detail. It is certainly worth further consideration in any future research.

Examples of Cases in the Research Study

Case 5C.[21] Boy aged 11 years 3 months and in July of 5th class in a private school in New South Wales, at the time of his original diagnostic appraisal session.

His father and mother were divorced and each of the divorced parents had further children to the new spouse. The brother and a half-brother of the boy (the father's son to the new marriage) also attended the clinic, the former partly concurrently with the client and the latter some years later.

At the interview with the mother that immediately preceded the diagnostic session, she informed the clinician that her son day-dreamed a lot, had frequent nightmares, was impulsive in much of his behaviour, stammered a little at times, and his school achievement was low.

She said that her son's "mind wanders" (poor concentration) and that was quickly verifiable when testing began. His memory was, not surprisingly, poor. He recognised that he was a problem both educationally and emotionally, and the family entanglements caused him a great deal of anxiety.

His I.Q. was 118 so that his reading lag of at least two years behind the expected *averages* for grade was in fact even greater than the scores indicated, as one would normally expect a boy of *above average* ability to perform at above average level. It should be noted also that he was older than would usually be expected for July of 5th class.

He showed marked fluctuations in level of performance in various tests and sub-tests, and typically "rushed" into a task, giving up or easing back very soon after the initial burst.

---

[21] Reference numbers are those used in the study.

He spent two years at the clinic (six terms of one 2-hour session per week), gradually overtaking the lag. He did not reach the *above average* level that one might hope for in his case, but he did bring his levels of performance to a range of between a year's lag behind grade expectancy on the A.C.E.R. Reading Tests and actual grade expectancy on occasion, with slight passing of grade expectancy once or twice.

There was a noticeable improvement in his emotional adjustment during this time, and his general school work, additional to his reading, showed improvement, according to school reports.

Four years after the completion of his remedial training in the clinic, the boy, now seventeen, visited me to discuss, quite maturely his plans to go on to further study when he left school. The Headmaster was pleased with his progress, although he still had some hard work to do if he was to achieve his plans in the years ahead.

He still expressed some concern about his parental difficulties, but without marked tension. He verbalised on the need to come to terms with this. He said that the period he spent in the reading clinic had helped him to settle down in general, and also had enabled him to pass examinations. Previously his record had been one of almost total failure. His plans for the future were realistic, and he had good insight into his limitations as well as an appreciation of his strengths—in contrast to his previous lack of self-confidence.

I had him come along for a few more "chats" to verbalise a little more about his domestic relationships and then suggested that he terminate the visits as there was good room for optimism regarding the eventual outcome of his emotional adjustment.

Case 6C. Boy, aged 9 years 1 month in grade 4B at a private school in New South Wales. He is half-brother of Case 5C above, having the same father. His family pattern is more stable than is the case with his two half-brothers as his mother and father are currently married to one another and he lives with them and their other children. His I.Q. score was 90, but the sub-test score pattern was markedly erratic, and a note was made on his diagnostic card that his true ability level was almost certainly higher, and on subsequent re-testing he obtained a score of 105.

His reading age was 8 years and 7 months but showed evidence also of the fluctuating levels of performance seen often by the author, as I have remarked in reading problem cases. In one area (individual recognition of words) he scored a little above grade expectancy. He was inclined to "rush" through work superficially and was not favourably disposed to checking over a test when he had gone through it, no matter how much time he had to spare.

His mother stated that she "thinks" his relations with other children at school are satisfactory, but he does not say much. Although he is not easily upset, and does not worry much, he is sometimes at loggerheads with his mother. The clinical observation of the boy together with an assessment of his test results and his test result profile indicated mild emotional tension whereas his half-brother 5C above has been marked as in definite need of psychological support. He was three terms (of one two-hour session per week) in the clinic and his daily record card showed mild but positive improvement in both his emotional adjustment and his reading performance. For instance, his original speed of reading (recorded after half a term in the clinic) was 103 words per minute on his comprehension tests; this had risen to 600 words per minute, despite more difficult levels of tests, after three terms, fluctuating on two occasions down to 194 words per minute and 200 words per minute. Earlier percentages ranged from 40 per cent to 90 and 100 per cent. Towards the end, scores were always 90 to 100 per cent, with 100 per cent predominating.

My reason for recording mild improvement only was some continuation of fluctuation up and down, on occasions.

Recorded comment here was: "His progress is most pleasing," and, although he obviously still had some way to go, he was showing evidence of ability to grapple with the situation himself, especially as he seemed more emotionally stable. The recommendation therefore (which was accepted) was that he terminate enrolment at the end of term, try progress on his own for a time, then, if need be, report back for refresher assistance. Since that time (two terms ago) there has been no opportunity as yet of following up the case further.

Case 7C. Boy aged 12 years and 3 months at time of diagnostic appraisal, first year of secondary school in a private school in Sydney. I.Q. 127 and reading retardation ranging from one to two years. He is the brother of No. 5C and half-brother of No. 6C above. He was about six months younger than the average boy in his class.

In the interview the mother described her son as "a worrier" and said that he had a history of asthma, and that until her re-marriage he was a bed-wetter. The records do not indicate when the re-marriage took place, but other entries suggest that it was about 3 years prior to the interview. Other comments by the mother were to the effect that the boy had a "strong sense of justice and right" and that he tried very hard at tasks, but was "impossible when tired".

It is readily apparent from this description of the boy that he was quite a deal more emotionally maladjusted than his half-brother, No. 6C, but more or less on a par with his full brother, No. 5C.

He is without a doubt a success story for remedial reading treatment. He was in the clinic for three and a half terms of one two-hour session per week and his record cards indicate continuous improvement to very satisfactory levels and comments about his increasing emotional adjustment are made. The best way of describing his success is to say that he has now gone on to a University and is reported to be happy and progressing favourably in his course there.

No. 5C, during his recent talk with me about his own proposed tertiary work, told me that his brother had come to terms with the domestic problem some time earlier and has made suggestions to No. 5C whereby he, too, might do so and generally adjust better.

THOSE WITH NO HISTORY OF READING PROBLEMS IN THE FAMILY

Case 106. Boy aged eight years and two months at time of diagnosis, and in third class in a private school in New South Wales. He was referred to us by a psychiatrist at the Children's Hospital to whom he had been referred for behaviour problems and for lack of adequate progress at school.

The mother was inclined to attempt domination of the clinician-parent interviews and would be unperturbed by late arrival for an appointment. She had rather firm ideas on what was wrong with the boy and often gave the impression that she was expressing her own values and opinions, but vicariously, using her son's name as the originator of these values. For example, her husband was the managing-director of a large manufacturing firm; she gave many evidences of class consciousness, and stated that the boy "has a definite attitude to rank or class of people and is accordingly proud of his father" or of his father's position.

"It matters to him that his father gives orders in his firm." The size of an institution was said to matter to the boy—the fact that the school he attended now, as against the school in a country town he had attended earlier, was "big" was important to him.

The mother stated that her son has been a "behaviour problem" for several years, both at home and at school. He "annoys his teachers intensely without their being able to say how or why. He is wayward and negativistic". He changed school several times in the short time since he commenced school, but without apparent improvement in his adjustment and progress. "All three previous schools have been glad to see him go."

It seemed to the mother that he may be "backward mentally", by which she presumably meant of poor intelligence. In fact, the boy scored 115 on the W.I.S.C. (Weschsler Intelligence Scale for Children) and 116 (later in the year) on the A.C.E.R. Junior Non-Verbal test. As one might expect, however, his results were erratic and he scored 105 on a Junior Non-Verbal Test on another occasion. He was averse to checking back over his completed tests even when he had ample time to do so.

The psychiatrist felt that there was some possibility of brain damage, both in view of his erratic test responses at times and the fact that he had had "a difficult birth".

On the "Illinois Test of Psycholinguistic Ability" he scored *above normal* on "motor-eye", "auditory-motor", and "auditory discrimination" with *problem* scores on the "visual motor sections" and on the "auditory verbal sections".

There are five children in the family and it is recorded that "he resented having a nurse help, when he was young".

He is right-handed, but fed left-handed at the outset.

The mother said that he was easily upset and she "thinks" he is a worrier—"over funny things", but did not elaborate on this.

The psychiatrist was of the opinion that the boy needed help from a male clinician (but accepted the fact that he would have to be assisted by a female in our clinic—my daughter—if he was to enter at the time). The teacher at school was a woman and "doesn't like him", but the mother was not surprised at this, as "he always drives women to tears" (including the mother). His mother had "longed for a son" but wondered whether perhaps the boy resented the happy relationship which she claimed, existed between the parents and whether this may have been the basis for the reading problem and emotional maladjustment in her son.

The psychiatrist was never able (or perhaps willing) to decide firmly on the possible minimal brain damage at birth.

His physical handling of cards and papers was "jerky", but this did not seem to result from any observable tremor of his hands, but to be the outcome of emotional tension when asked to give his attention to a particular task, and at times to be an attempt to "see how far he could go" with disruptive behaviour. In other words he would become *physically* steadier, as well as less noisy and more attentive to explanations and requests if they were given reasonably firmly.

His Reading Retardation was in the order of 18 months below expected *average* for his age, but, as pointed out above, he was of *above average* ability. His attack on fundamentals—phonetic analysis and synthesis of words—was poor.

Eighteen months after he entered the clinic (where he remained for 6 terms of one two-hour session per week) his reading levels on A.C.E.R. tests had risen to *above average* for his age and grade and his behaviour was closer to normal. It was found that the "father-to-son" line with this boy, firm but kindly, was productive of good results all round in the clinic, as had been noticed above in the testing session. I told him that neither he nor I nor anyone else can be allowed to disrupt the welfare of other people, and took the step of placing him with a group of older boys who would not look kindly on disruptive behaviour in him. He made a quite marked upward movement in level of school work and in behaviour—even topping his class in English.

Of the four siblings of this boy (three sisters and one brother) one was reported to be "usually in an A form", two as "satisfactory at school" and one was only four years old.

Case 120. Girl aged 15 years and 2 months, I.Q. 120, lagging approximately one and one half years behind the achievement expectancy for a student of her personal ability level. This was an estimate made by the clinician at the time of the diagnostic appraisal. There are no school records appended to the diagnostic papers, but on information provided at the interview with the parent, a note was made that her school work (English 51 per cent, French 78 per cent, Biology 57 per cent, General Mathematics 68 per cent, Modern History 78 per cent, Economics 70 per cent) bears out this estimate of eighteen months lag. It was also noted that some tension was evident, mainly in the erratic nature of her scoring profile, but as no other information supporting slight tension is recorded, she has been marked "nil" for the presence of emotional maladjustment.

This is in keeping with my personal opinion of the girl from observation in the clinic subsequent to the diagnostic appraisal. Also it is recorded that the mother stated that her daughter is not easily upset and that, outwardly at any rate, she was not a worrier—"except at examination times". She was also stated to be neither over-aggressive nor over-submissive in the presence of her peers.

Her young brother (her only sibling) was seven years of age at the time she was tested. It is recorded that he was progressing "quite well" at school and that she was on quite good terms with him, but "picks on him a bit" now and again. She was a pupil at a private girls' secondary school. (Any non-state school is termed "private" for the purpose of this book—both Catholic and non-Catholic.)

The mother's estimate of the girl's progress, "reports always good", do not correspond very well with the results gained in examinations, unless the school was rather more kindly in remarks on her report than schools usually are. The school may have been of the opinion that her ability was lower than the 120 given above (she measured down to 106 on another I.Q. test here on another occasion during one of the swings in level of performance), and perhaps considered that she was therefore measuring up fairly well to the expectancy level of a "bright normal".

The girl described her spelling proficiency as "medium".

The estimate of "considerable" reading improvement was made on the progress recorded on her daily work card (she was in the clinic for ten 2-hour sessions, one per day, five days per week, for two weeks). Her speed of reading, both on the comprehension exercises and on the narrative reading on the reading machine progressed consistently and with increasing gains from 308 words per minute to 2031 (machine) and 2143 (timed comprehension exercises). I realise that research is going on at the present time on the reliability and validity of comprehension test scores in reading, but I have no reason to reject scores obtained by this girl or those obtained by anyone else. They were mainly 80 per cent to 100 per cent, 50 per cent on one occasion, 56 per cent on another, 63 per cent and 67 per cent on other occasions (once each) and a couple of times in the 70s; as she increased her speed of reading, she also increased the difficulty level of the material read.

The girl was personally pleased with her progress.

Case 136. A girl of sixteen years and eight months, I.Q. 121, who spent two terms in the clinic. She was a pupil at a private school in New South Wales. She was in 5th year of secondary school. She considered that she read too slowly and it was stated by her mother during the interview that the girl did not read much for pleasure, even allowing for the fact that no-one has a great deal of time to read for pleasure in the matriculation examination year.

Her speed score at the time of diagnosis was 300 words per minute, and at the time of completion of her period in the clinic 800 words per minute on her comprehension tests and 1545 on her machine reading (narrative material). She is recorded as having achieved mild reading improvement because it was not until the end of her first term in the clinic that she raised her speed to 454, then 461, 686 and 720 words per minute on her last four tests for the term and there was less consistency in the raising of difficulty levels than, for example, with Case 136. Her comprehension scores, except for one 50 per cent and one or two 60s and 70s were mainly 80 per cent and 100 per cent and her vocabulary was at the expected level.

The girl herself made the original appointment with me and the general family opinion (including the girl's) as reported to me was that reading help would be a means of "reliancy development". As she was one of the most *reliable* girls I had enrolled in the clinic I was not entirely sure of how to construe the "reliancy development" concept. It subsequently turned out to mean that her "risk" of failure in her goals (and the family's goals) in her educational endeavours, would be decreased.

Friends at school who felt that they had benefited from reading assistance in this clinic had recommended that she come here. She seemed to me to have made a mature judgment and was following it through. She gave no impression of emotional maladjustment, except perhaps that I should like to have seen her a little less all-absorbed in her attempt at achievement in tasks to which she applied herself.

She was described as "sensitive", but not too easily upset, "an extrovert, completely, in a group of friends", but she was reported as a "worrier". This latter characteristic—if it was a characteristic of her—was not observable to any marked degree in the clinic, unless the absorption with successful outcome of tasks in hand was slight evidence of this.

The final letter or "report" that I sent to her father contains some phrases that sum up both the girl as I saw her, and the progress she had made. I said that she had done well (and gave reasons for this assessment) and added that "she has been a very pleasant person to have here".

After consideration of all the relevant factors she was given a "nil" evaluation with reference to emotional maladjustment.

CONCLUSION

From the material that has been presented in this book, it is clear that while there is a current ferment over dyslexia, many advances have been reported in the past decade or so as a result of this interest. It is also clear, however, that the problem of reading disability, congenital or otherwise, has been a matter of major concern to educationalists and psychologists, and to a lesser extent, medical practitioners, for a long time. No doubt the intensified emphasis on the importance of education in the modern technological world, both to the individual and to society (nationally and internationally) has been responsible for some of the increased interest in the topic.

It has been claimed that reading is the key to success in all subjects—given sufficient ability, drive, educational opportunity, health and intellectual curiosity in the individual. Certainly, the claim has more than an element of truth in it. In the days of a lower school leaving age, and less demand (or opportunity) for graduates of tertiary (especially university) institutions, a reading disability would have been an almost insurmountable barrier to ambition; the dyslexic would have left school as soon as possible and teachers or parents would have felt little need to spend undue time worrying over him.

But today, with our overcrowded classrooms and university entrance quotas, the problem is there for all to see and is a matter of general concern. Happily, by one approach or another, assistance *is* being given to many who would otherwise fall by the way, and this trend will without doubt continue and accelerate. True, the educationally retarded is still, too often, left to his own devices by an understandably harassed teacher overwhelmed by sheer weight of numbers. However, at least the *need* for assistance is now being recognised. When problems of finance, teacher shortage and administration are overcome or reduced, advances in understanding and in method will considerably relieve the plight of the psychologically and educationally disabled child, to the advantage of himself and the community as a whole.

BIBLIOGRAPHY

As a help to readers in particular who are students of Education or Psychology and whose interest in the topic of dyslexia and remedial reading problems may lead them to further study or research in some aspect of this field, I have decided to include a wider bibliography than would normally be the case. No bibliography of course is exhaustive, but the following references have proved both interesting and useful to me in preparing this book and in carrying out my research on the topic of the effects of familial influence and emotional maladjustment on reading problems. One has only to glance at the reference lists appended to many of the papers presented at the 1968 Melbourne Dyslexia Symposium to realise how many additional sources might be consulted, although, of course, there is quite a deal of overlap of hard-core references in all lists concerned with this problem.

The vast extent of the literature on reading is highlighted by Alfredo Namnum and Ernst Prelinger (1961) who refer to Betts and Betts' *Index to Professional Literature on Reading and Related Topics,* which covered publications up to the year 1943, but unfortunately is not annotated. It contains 8,278 entries. They mention also the three reviews by Traxler of *Research on Reading,* which covers the period from 1930 to 1953, in which although admittedly incomplete, have been catalogued and abstracted 1,905 references. There are 434 references concerning reading for the years 1954 to 1958, and yet their listing overlaps only partially those in the annual summaries by W. S. Gray in the *Journal of Educational Research.* Namnum and Prelinger point out that this means that at least 2,500 publications relevant to the field of reading have been made in the thirty years prior to 1961. To this number must be added the very substantial number of papers and books on one aspect or another of reading, including reading disability, published since that date.

ARTHUR, Grace: "Tutoring and Remedial Teaching as Educational Therapy", in *Readings in the Clinical Method in Psychology* (ed. R. I. Watson), Harper & Brothers, New York, 1949.
ATKINSON, Joan K.: Reading Improvement Through Psycholinguistic Remediation—*The Slow Learning Child,* 1967, *14,* 2.

ATKINSON, Joan K.; COCHRANE, Kathleen J.; and ELKINS, J.: Retarded Readers at High School Start—An Investigation in Diagnosis and Treatment—*The Slow Learning Child,* 1968, *15,* 2.

ATKINSON, Joan K.: Diagnostic Therapy and Remedial Teaching—*Proceedings, Dyslexia Symposium, Melbourne,* The Australian College of Speech Therapists, Melbourne, 1968.

BANNATYNE, A. D.: The Aetiology of Dyslexia—*The Slow Learning Child,* 1966, *13,* 1.

BARBER, B. J.: The Educational Problem—*Proceedings, Dyslexia Symposium, Melbourne,* The Australian College of Speech Therapists, Melbourne, 1968.

BLANCHARD, Phyllis: Reading Disabilities in Relation to Maladjustment—*Mental Hygiene,* 1928, *XII.*

BLANCHARD, Phyllis: "Tommy Nolan", in *Psychiatric Interviews With Children* (ed. Helen Leland Witmer), The Commonwealth Fund, New York, 1946.

BLANCHARD, Phyllis: Psychoanalytic Contributions to the Problems of Reading Disabilities—*The Psychoanalytic Study of the Child,* 1946, *2.*

BLATCH, Mary B.: Acquired Dyslexia—*Proceedings, Dyslexia Symposium, Melbourne,* The Australian College of Speech Therapists, Melbourne, 1968.

BURT, J. G.: *The Subnormal Mind,* Oxford University Press, London, 1935.

CLARK, B. T.: We Teach the Slow Learner to Read—*The Slow Learning Child,* 1964, *10,* 3.

CRITCHLEY, Macdonald: *Developmental Dyslexia,* William Heinemann Medical Books Limited, London, 1964.

CRITCHLEY, Macdonald: Is Developmental Dyslexia the Expression of Minor Cerebral Damage?—*The Slow Learning Child,* 1966, *13,* 1.

COLVIN, J.: Opthalmological Aspects of Developmental Dyslexia—*Proceedings, Dyslexia Symposium, Melbourne,* The Australian College of Speech Therapists, Melbourne, 1968.

COOPER, J. L.: An Adaptation of the Fernald-Keller Approach to Teaching an Initial Reading Vocabulary to Children with Severe Reading Disabilities—*The Slow Learning Child,* 1964, *10,* 3.

DELLA-PIANA, G. M.: *Reading Diagnosis and Prescription,* Holt, Rinehart and Winston, Inc., New York, 1968.

DOLCH, E. W.: *Problems in Reading,* The Garrard Press, Champaign, 1948.

DOWNING, J. and BROWN, Amy L.: *The Second International Reading Symposium,* Cassell, London, 1967.

EAMES, T. H.: A Comparison of the Ocular Characteristics of Unselected and Reading Disability Groups—*Journal of Educational Research,* 1932, *25.*

FABIAN, A. A.: Reading Disability: An Index of Pathology—*American Journal of Orthopsychiatry,* 1955, *25.*

FERNALD, Grace M.: *Remedial Techniques in Basic School Subjects,* McGraw Hill Book Co., Inc., New York, 1943.

FROSTIG, Marianne: A Scale for the Evaluation of Movement Skills and a Programme of Sensory Motor Training—*Proceedings, Dyslexia Symposium, Melbourne,* The Australian College of Speech Therapists, Melbourne, 1968.

FROSTIG, Marianne: Remedial Reading Methods in Relation to Disabilities in Perception, Language and Thought Processes—*Proceedings, Dyslexia Symposium, Melbourne,* The Australian College of Speech Therapists, Melbourne, 1968.

FROSTIG, Marianne: Theory and Research Findings Concerning Learning Disturbances—*Proceedings, Dyslexia Symposium, Melbourne,* The Australian College of Speech Therapists, Melbourne, 1968.

GANN, Edith: *Reading Difficulty and Personality Organisation,* King's Crown Press, New York, 1945.

GATES, A. I.: *The Psychology of Reading and Spelling; with Special Reference to Disabilities,* Teachers' College, Columbia University, New York, 1922.

GATES, A. I. and BENNETT, C. C.: *Reversal Tendencies in Reading,* Bureau of Publications, Teachers' College, Columbia University, New York, 1933.

GATES, A. I. and BOND, G. L.: Relation of Handedness, Eyesighting and Acuity Dominance to Reading—*Journal of Educational Psychology,* 1936, *27.*

GATES, A. I. and BOND, G. L.: Reading Readiness. A Study of Factors Determining Success and Failure in Beginning to Read—*Teachers' College Record,* 1936, *37.*

GATES, A. I.: The Role of Personality Maladjustment in Reading Disability—*Journal of Genetic Psychology,* 1941, *LIX.*

GATES, A. I.: *The Improvement of Reading: A Program of Diagnostic and Remedial Methods,* The Macmillan Company, New York, 1947.

HALLGREN, Bertil: Specific Dyslexia (Congenital Word Blindness)— *Acta Psychiatrica et Neurologica, Supplementum 65,* Munksgaard, Copenhagen, 1950.

HARRIS, A. J.: *How to Increase Reading Ability,* David McKay Company, Inc., New York, 1961.

HART, N.: The Early Diagnosis and Treatment of Children with Psycholinguistic Difficulties—*Proceedings, Dyslexia Symposium, Melbourne,* The Australian College of Speech Therapists, Melbourne, 1968.

HERMANN, Knud: *A Medical Study of Word-Blindness and Related Handicaps,* Munksgaard, Copenhagen, 1959.

HINSHELWOOD, J.: Congenital Word-Blindness, with Reports of Two Cases—*Oph. Rev.,* 1902, *21.*

HINSHELWOOD, J.: *Congenital Word Blindness,* H. K. Lewis & Co., London, 1917.

HOGAN, T. K.: Nomograph for Tetrachoric Correlation—*Australian Journal of Psychology*, 1949, *1*, 1.

HOOPER, Freda and HARRISON, R. N. (Ed.): *Proceedings, Dyslexia Symposium, Melbourne*, The Australian College of Speech Therapists, Melbourne, 1968.

HOOPER, Freda: Statement of the Problem of Dyslexia—*Proceedings, Dyslexia Symposium, Melbourne*, The Australian College of Speech Therapists, Melbourne, 1968.

HOPKINS, I.: Neurological Assessment of Children with Special Reference to Dyslexia—*Proceedings, Dyslexia Symposium, Melbourne*, The Australian College of Speech Therapists, Melbourne, 1968.

INGLIS, W. B.: "The Early Stages of Reading: A Review of Recent Investigations"—in *Studies in Reading*, University of London Press, for the Scottish Council for Research in Education, London, 1968.

ISAACS, Susan: "The Nature and Function of Phantasy"—in *Developments in Psychoanalysis*, Klein et al, Hillary House, New York, 1952.

JOHNSON, Marjorie: Factors Related to Disability in Reading—*Journal of Experimental Education*, 1957, *XXVI*, 1.

JAMESON, A.: "Methods and Devices for Remedial Reading"—in *Recent Trends in Reading* (edited by W. S. Gray)—*Supplementary Educational Monographs, No. 49*, University of Chicago Press, 1939.

KLEIN, Melanie: *Our Adult World and Its Roots in Infancy*, Tavistock Publications, London, 1960.

KLEIN, Melanie: A Note on Depression in the Schizophrenic—*International Journal of Psycho-Analysis*, 1960, *XVI*.

LYLE, J. G.: Some Psychological Factors in Reading Retardation—*Australian Journal of Psychology*, 1954, *6*, 2.

McLAUGHLIN, R. M.: *Schizoid Dyslexia*—M.A. Thesis, University of N.S.W., 1965.

McLEOD, J.: Prediction of Childhood Dyslexia—*The Slow Learning Child*, 1966, *12*, 3.

McLEOD, J.: From Labels to Action—*The Slow Learning Child*, 1967, *14*, 2.

McLEOD, J.: *Dyslexia Schedule*, University of Queensland Press, Brisbane, 1969.

McLEOD, J.: *Handbook for Dyslexia Schedule and School Entrance Check List*, University of Queensland Press, Brisbane, 1969.

McLEOD, J.: *School Entrance Check List*, University of Queensland Press, Brisbane, 1969.

McNEMARR, Q.: *Psychological Statistics*, John Wiley and Sons Inc., New York and London, Third Edition, 1962.

MEEHL, P. E.: A Reformulation of the Problem of Reading Disability—*Journal of Child Psychiatry*, 1956, *3*.

MEEHL, P. E.: Schizotaxia, Schizotypy, Schizophrenia—*American Psychologist*, 1962, *17*, 12.

MONEY, J.: Learning Disability and the Principles of Reading—*The Slow Learning Child*, 1967, *14*, 2.

MONEY, J. (Ed.): *The Disabled Reader, Education of the Dyslexic Child*, The Johns Hopkins Press, Baltimore, 1966.

MONROE, Marion: *Children Who Cannot Read*, University of Chicago Press, Chicago, 1932.

MONROE, Marion and BACKUS, B.: *Remedial Reading: A Monograph in Character Education*, Houghton Mifflin Co., Boston, 1937.

MORGAN, W. P.: A Case of Congenital Word-Blindness—*British Medical Journal*, 1896, *II*.

MYKLEBUST, Helena R. and JOHNSON, Doris: Dyslexia in Children—*Exceptional Children*, 1962.

NAMNUM, A. and PRELINGER, E.: On the Psychology of the Reading Process—*American Journal of Orthopsychiatry*, 1961, *31*.

NEALE, Marie D.: Patterns of Dyslexia. Predictive Studies of Dyslexia and Early Intervention—*Proceedings, Dyslexia Symposium, Melbourne*, The Australian College of Speech Therapists, Melbourne, 1968.

NEWALL, N.: For Non-Readers in Distress — *Elementary School Journal*, 1931, *32*.

NURCOMBE, B.: Learnıng Disability and Emotional Disorder—*The Slow Learning Child*, 1967, *14*, 2.

ORTON, S. T.: A Neurological Explanation of Reading Disability—*Educational Record*, 1931, *XX*.

ORTON, S. T.: *Reading, Writing and Speech Problems in Children*—Norton & Co., New York, 1937.

PEARSON, G.: A Survey of Learning Difficulties in Children—*The Psychoanalytic Study of The Child*, 1952, *7*.

POSTMAN, L. (Ed.): *Psychology in the Making*, Alfred A. Knopf, New York, 1964.

PRESCOTT, D. A.: *Emotion and the Educative Process*, American Council on Education, Washington, 1938.

PRESTON, M. J.: Reading Failure and the Child's Security—*American Journal of Orthopsychiatry*, 1940, *10*.

RICKARDS, W. S.: Emotional Problems of the Dyslexic Child—*Proceedings, Dyslexia Symposium, Melbourne*, The Australian College of Speech Therapists, Melbourne, 1968.

ROBINSON, H.: *Why Pupils Fail in Reading*, University of Chicago Press, Chicago, 1946.

SAUNDERS, R. E.: Dyslexia: More Than Reading Retardation—*The Slow Learning Child*, 1965, *11*, No. 3.

SCHONELL, F. J.: *Backwardness in the Basic Subjects*, Oliver and Boyd, Edinburgh, 1948.

SCHONELL, F. J.: *Diagnostic and Attainment Testing*, Oliver and Boyd, Edinburgh, 1950.

SHAW, Edna: The Philosophy of Dr. Gattegno and Its Implication for an Experiment in Literacy—*Proceedings, Dyslexia Symposium, Melbourne,* The Australian College of Speech Therapists, Melbourne, 1968.

SILVERMAN, R.; FITE, J.; and MOSHER, P.: Learning Problems, *I*: Clinical findings in reading disability children; special cases of intellectual inhibition—*American Journal of Orthopsychiatry,* 1959, *29.*

SMITH, Nila B.: Research on Reading and the Emotions—*School and Society,* 1955, *81.*

STRACHEY, J.: Some Unconscious Factors in Reading—*International Journal of Psycho-Analysis,* 1930, *XI.*

SYLVESTER, E. and KUNST, M.: Psychodynamic Aspects of the Reading Problem—*American Journal of Orthopsychiatry,* 1943, *13.*

TAMKIN, A. S.: A Survey of Educational Disability in Emotionally Disturbed Children—*Journal of Educational Research,* 1960, *54.*

TOMATIS, A.: *Dyslexia,* McGraw Hill, New York, 1968.

TOMATIS, A.: The Basis of Dyslexia—*Journal of Applied Psychology,* 1968, *1.*

TOMATIS, A.: *Dyslexia,* University of Ottawa Press, Ottawa, 1969. Translated by Dr. A. Sidlauskas.

THORNDIKE, R. L.: *Personnel Selection, Test and Measurement Techniques,* John Wiley and Sons, Inc., New York, 1949.

TULCHIN, S. H.: Emotional Factors in Reading Disabilities in School Children—*Journal of Educational Psychology,* 1935, *26.*

VERNON, Magdalen Dorothea: *Backwardness in Reading; a Study of Its Nature and Origin,* University Press, Cambridge, 1957.

VERNON, Magdalen Dorothea: Specific Dyslexia—*The Slow Learning Child,* 1965, *12, 2.*

WILKING, S. V.: Personality Maladjustment as a Causative Factor in Reading Disability—*Elementary School Journal,* 1941, *42.*

WITTY, P. and KOPEL, D.: Sinistral and Mixed Manual-Ocular Behaviour in Reading Disability—*Journal of Educational Psychology,* 1936, *XXVII.*